INSTRUCTIONS
HOW TO FILL OUT
THE *BEAT THE ODDS*
HEALTH QUESTIONNAIRE

Start with a #2 pencil

- Print your name and address on page one.
- Fill in responses only within the ovals.
- Erase wrong answers completely.
- Review your completed questionnaire to make sure you have answered all the questions you can.
- If you don't know the answers to questions about blood pressure, cholesterol, and high-density lipoprotein (HDL), ask your physician or leave these areas blank. If you leave them blank, the average values for your age, race, and sex will be used to prepare your health profile. It is far preferable to provide proper answers.

Be sure to answer the following questions

You *must* answer the following questions so that General Health Inc. can process your report and send it to you.

- Name and address
- 1.00 Sex
- 1.01 Age
- 1.02 Weight
- 1.03 Height
- 3.06 Race or Ethnic Background

Some questions touch on very personal subjects, but for a very good reason—because the answers let us tell you about your health risks. For example, white Anglo-Saxon men have a higher rate of prostate cancer than Jewish men. That's one reason for the questions on race and religion.

Your personalized *Beat the Odds Health Profile* will be produced by comparing your questionnaire responses to data for people of your age, sex, physical characteristics, and race or ethnic background. Without that basic information, General Health Inc. cannot provide you with an accurate report on your health risks.

When you are finished

- Copy your identification number from the front of the questionnaire here:

  _____

- Write in the date you mailed the questionnaire here: _____
- Mail the questionnaire, unfolded, in the enclosed prepaid envelope, along with a check for $10.00 made out to General Health Inc., to:

  General Health Inc.
  3299 K Street, N.W.
  Washington, D.C 20007

Confidentiality guaranteed

General Health Inc. will maintain the confidentiality of your answers. General Health Inc. will not permit any personally identifiable information from your health data record to be obtained by any person or organization at any time for any reason whatsoever without first obtaining your written permission. Of course, we cannot be responsible for improper or unauthorized uses of information in your *BTO Questionnaire* and/or *BTO Profile* if you share this information with others or participate in a program in which you permit others to handle the *BTO Questionnaire* and/or *BTO Profile.*

Questions

If you have any questions about your *BTO Questionnaire* or *BTO Profile,* call General Health Inc. at (800) 424-2775 during East Coast business hours. In the Washington, D.C., area, call 965-4881.

Limitation of liability

Any *Beat the Odds Health Profile* demonstrated to be in error solely as a result of General Health Inc. processing shall be reprocessed. This is, however, your only remedy, and General Health Inc. and Villard Books specifically disclaim responsibility and liability for any other damages arising out of or in connection with your use of the *BTO Health Profile* whether based on contract or tort. In no event shall General Health Inc. or Villard Books be liable for any consequential or special damages which you may incur. By submitting your *Beat the Odds Health Questionnaire* for processing, you are agreeing to be bound by the above limitation of liability.

Beat the Odds and the *Beat the Odds Health Profile* are not meant to replace your doctor or substitute for medical care. They are to be used in consultation with your doctor.

The *BTO Profile* is not designed to give you a diagnosis of illness or a prediction about an individual's health. A statement about risk is not a prediction about you, the *individual.* Statements about your risk are about the likelihood of an event like death or illness occurring in a group of people with or without a certain set of characteristics just like yours. Given your specific data, the *BTO Profile* will not tell you something that *will* happen, but what the odds are that it *may* happen.

The *BTO Profile* is also *not designed:*

• to assess your risks of dying from a condition you already have
• to be used by people under 20 or over 74
• to tell you specifically how to change your behavior. Once you know what your risks are, you can use your local resources to help improve your health.

Beat
the Odds

Beat the Odds

HAROLD S. SOLOMON, M.D.,
with
LAWRENCE D. CHILNICK

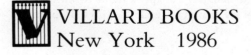 VILLARD BOOKS
New York   1986

Grateful acknowledgment is made to the following for permission to reprint previously published material:

American Cancer Society: a chart which appeared in an American Cancer Society report on cancer related check-ups. (1980; 30:194–240.) Reprinted by permission.

Bantam Books, Inc.: excerpts from *The Little Black Pill Book,* Lawrence D. Chilnick, editor-in-chief. Copyright © 1983 by The Food and Drug Book Company, Inc.; excerpts from *Pill Book of High Blood Pressure,* Lawrence D. Chilnick, editor-in-chief. Copyright © 1985 by The Food and Drug Book Company, Inc. Reprinted by permission of Bantam Books, Inc. All rights reserved.

The Berkley Publishing Group: Six charts from *The Cokebook* by Larry Chilnick and Bert Stern. Copyright © 1984 by Bookmark Books, Inc. Reprinted by permission of The Berkley Publishing Group.

Facts on File Publications: Two charts, which were adapted from *Riskwatch* by John Urquhart and Klaus Heilman. © 1984 by Kindler Verlag, GmbH. Reprinted with permission of Facts on File, Inc., New York.

86-40098
ISBN 0-394-55286-5
ISBN 0-394-75350-X (pbk.)

Text design by Levavi & Levavi
Manufactured in the United States of America
9 8 7 6 5 4 3 2
First Edition

Dedicated to my teachers: My grandparents and parents, my wife and children, George Parthemos, Thomas Brittingham, David Rodgers, and Eugene Braunwald—and, of course, my patients.

H.S.

Beat the Odds and the *Beat the Odds Health Profile* are not meant to replace your doctor or substitute for medical care. They are to be used in consultation with your doctor.

The *BTO Profile* is not designed to give you a diagnosis of illness or a prediction about an individual's health. A statement about risk is not a prediction about you, the *individual*. Statements about your risk are about the likelihood of an event like death or illness occurring in a group of people with or without a certain set of characteristics just like yours. Given your specific data, the *BTO Profile* will not tell you something that *will* happen, but what the odds are that it *may* happen.

The *BTO Profile* is also *not designed:*

- to assess your risks of dying from a condition you already have
- to be used by people under 20 or over 74
- to tell you specifically how to change your behavior. Once you know what your risks are, you can use your local resources to help improve your health.

Acknowledgments

Over the course of the past two years, many dedicated colleagues and friends have contributed in numerous ways to *Beat the Odds*. Without their assistance, insight, and constructive criticism, our task would have been considerably more difficult.

We are especially grateful to Daniel Montopoli for his research expertise and his invaluable contribution to several chapters in the book, which benefited enormously from his talents.

The staff of General Health Inc., who participated in the creation of this book from its inception to its conclusion, have assisted us continually. They include James L. Bernstein, M.D.; Dan Klein; Jean Duff; and Axel Goetz, who helped us see this book through to its fruition.

Our gratitude is also extended to our colleagues at the Healthstyle Program, including Howard Hartley, M.D.; Fran Raab; Alan Herd, M.D.; and Bernard Howes, D.D.S., who helped form that program, which is the inspiration for *Beat the Odds*.

Others whose unique professional abilities contributed to this book are Marc Jaffe, Peter Gethers, Laura Godfrey, Linda Rosenberg, and Ruth Randall at Villard Books. In addition, Julie Surrey, Bert Stern, Jay Acton, Ned Leavitt, and Mark S. Gold, M.D., provided timely and deft critical judgments, for which we are grateful.

Contents

Preface: Disease and Your Risks

When we started writing this book, our premise was simple: People who know their health risks, learn about disease prevention, and have a good relationship with a trusted physician, can beat the odds and live longer.

We also felt that most of the popular medical self-care books promised unrealistic, generalized "quick fixes" that really didn't work, because each person's health problems are different. How, then, could we write a book that would really help you to improve your odds of living longer and lower your risk of future illness?

To solve this, we have created what we think is the world's first interactive health book. Everyone who buys this book should first complete the *Beat the Odds Health Questionnaire* (see the opening pages of this book for instructions) and then mail it in to be processed and analyzed against the giant data base of General Health Inc.'s health risk appraisal program. You will then receive a computer-generated report, the *Beat the Odds Health Profile*, which will contain very specific information about your own individual health risks. With this report, you will be directed to specific sections of this book, which contains all the information you need to know in order to reduce specific health risks and beat the odds.

Basically, this book is divided into two sections.

Chapters One to Twelve recommend specific strategies for the prevention of disease. But even if you take advantage of all these strategies, we think it's important to go beyond that information. So, we thought, why not add to the book some information about commonly occurring illnesses, which will add directly to the knowledge of the reader? And as long as we were doing this, why not call upon trusted clinical colleagues who had proved their skills over and over again with patients referred to them. The reader benefits from their good opinion and judgment, just as their patients do.

Therefore, we have assembled the second section of the book directly from information supplied by expert colleagues in Boston.

In Chapters Thirteen to Twenty-two, we present information on many common ailments, some of which are not preventable because we don't yet have the knowledge to do this. But an informed patient can always be treated more effectively. By understanding your disease, you can maximize your potential for treatment.

We believe that we've presented the most important facts in a succinct, comprehensible manner. We don't feel that patients have to be medical students in order to understand more about their disease, and we do believe that patients should know more than they can be told in a brief office visit. The material is designed to be an overview.

The following people have assisted us in this section: cancer: Graham Coldizt, M.D., M.B.B.S., Research Associate in Medicine, Channing Laboratory, Brigham and Women's Hospital and Harvard Medical School; respiratory disease: Christopher Fanta, M.D., Assistant Professor of Medicine, Harvard Medical School, Director of Pulmonary Consultant Bronchoscopy Services, Brigham and Women's Hospital; muscular/skeletal conditions: Jonathan S. Coblyn, M.D., Assistant Professor of Medicine, Harvard Medical School, and Associate Physician and Director, Rheumatology Consultant Service, Brigham and Women's Hospital; gastrointestinal disorders: Richard Curtis, M.D., Instructor in Medicine, Tufts University, and Attending Physician, New England Baptist and Newton-Wellesley hospitals; neurology: Martin A. Samuels, M.D., Associate Professor of Neurology, Harvard Medical School, Chief Neurology Service, V.A. Medical Center, Brockton–West Roxbury, Massachusetts; urology and reproduction: Gary P. Kearney, M.D., Clinical Associate Professor of Surgery, and Isaac Schiff, M.D., Associate Professor, Obstetrics and Gynecology, Harvard Medical School, and Associate Director, Reproductive Endocrinology, Brigham and Women's Hospital; exercise: Robert Goldszer, M.D., Harvard Medical School, Brigham and Women's Hospital; and accidents: Susan Scavo Gallagher, M.P.H., Director, Injury Prevention, Massachusetts Department of Public Health.

These later chapters may be referred to in your *Beat the Odds Health Profile*, even though some of the information they contain does not deal specifically with risk reduction.

We hope that you will not only read those sections of *Beat the Odds* that deal with your own medical risks, but will also refer to the rest of the information in the book, using it as a guide to a longer, healthier life-style.

HAROLD S. SOLOMON, M.D.
LAWRENCE D. CHILNICK

Beat
the Odds

Don't Gamble with Your Health!

THE STORY OF SILVER FOX THE BOOKIE

Why do some people beat the odds and live longer, healthier lives, while others do not?

Sometimes a simple identification of personal risk is all that's needed to make people change their health habits; sometimes it's finding just the right "trigger" that will motivate a certain type of person. For some people, simply showing them how high their risk is—giving them the necessary information—can be motivation enough. For others, it takes hitting the right emotional spark.

One of my most memorable patients was a "bookie" in his early fifties. He made his living gambling—it was the only work he had ever known—and had a totally disordered life-style. I found him to have an elevated cholesterol level and a strong family history of diabetes. He smoked too much, and he was twenty to thirty pounds overweight. In addition, he had rather severe high blood pressure, 160 over 115. I was concerned because he seemed to be on the verge of a very serious heart attack yet was not responding to my pleas that he change his "health habits." In desperation, I took out a Framingham risk chart, which is somewhat like the computer report you will be using in conjunction with this book. I showed him what the *average* likelihood was of having a heart attack over the next six years for someone his age, race, and sex. The chart showed that his risk was *triple* that of the average person of his age.

Over the next six months, The Silver Fox, as he called himself, fooled me. He lost weight, quit smoking, changed his behavior patterns, and lowered his blood pressure. One year after he began treatment, he came into my office as a model patient, and I really couldn't understand it.

"You know," I said to him, "I'm puzzled. I know about behavioral change, and you are one of the least likely people I've ever met to make these changes. Yet here you are and you've done everything you had to do."

He said, "Doc, I don't know from heart attacks and strokes, but remember that little booklet you showed me when I was in your office? That's what caused me to make all these changes. *I know from odds and I didn't like my odds!*"

You never know who is going to be a successful patient. A good physician is aware of certain things that may stand in the way of success, and the doctor should try to eliminate these obstacles. For example, lengthening one's life may not be important to a patient who is severely depressed. So before a doctor can begin to help such a patient make changes in health habits, that depression must be dealt with. People who have alcoholism masking an underlying condition may not reduce their drinking risk until the condition is under control. Doctors who deliver authoritarian lectures about being overweight are likely to have some patients drop out of care; these patients do not comply with the doctor's instructions because they can't handle *orders*, or find the doctor's tone too judgmental.

So, the doctor who sets out to help you reduce health risks today also has to be in tune with you and your nature as a patient, bringing into play all his or her motivational skills. This is one of the most crucial tasks facing medical professionals in the 1980s. It's also the reason we've created *Beat the Odds*. If we can motivate you to work with your doctor—if you can use this book to help your doctor understand you better—then we have succeeded!

KNOW YOUR HEALTH RISKS

Good health isn't something you *add* to your life. It is a way of life. Practicing good health is a lifelong activity involving behavior, life-style, and even environment. It is the most worthwhile activity you can undertake. Protecting your health will extend your life.

The way people choose to lead their lives—how they confront potential health hazards—dramatically affects their future health. Ironically, changing various *known* health hazards by reducing risk ahead of time has not been a high priority in this country. Almost 20 percent of our health-care budget is spent on people in the last months of their lives, while barely 2 percent is spent on all preventive health-care activities. By accepting these priorities, we have acknowledged that the medical establishment's primary job is only to "practice medicine." It is up to the *individual* to be responsible for his or her own physical well-being and for the prevention of illness.

Of course, it is important to remember that although medicine has focused for years on the problems of illness rather than preventive health care, such developments as new types of vaccinations, better sterile surgical techniques, modern medical treatment facilities, and increased sanitation have improved overall health. Obviously, prevention is not more or less important than the "high-tech" aspects of medicine. The balance of the two is what's crucial.

We no longer worry about the health problems that plagued our grandparents' generation, mostly infections. The diseases we've developed from stress, from our environment, and from too much food, alcohol, and tobacco are now the main focus of medical care. There is a whole range of diseases directly related to modern life-styles. In fact, more people die of life-style-related illnesses, such as heart attacks, than of diseases caused by a viral or bacterial infection.

Yet, we put off seeing a doctor until we are sick. People still use doctors to keep from getting sicker, rather than using them to *prevent* illness. To meet the increasing range of life-style-related diseases, physicians have evolved a system that emphasizes *diagnosis* and *treatment* of ongoing symptoms or identified disease. The basic goal of current medical practice is to find a cure for—or, at the very least, to identify—the problem. Until recently, preventive health care was often a secondary function of the family doctor and/or the specialist, if they did any health educating at all.

Medicine has been slow to recognize its new role in an age in which disease is related to the patient's health practices. Even if you do go for a checkup, a typical visit to a family physician finds the patient sitting across from the doctor, quickly answering questions about medical history, then undergoing a brief exam and some blood or urine tests. If, later, the test results show elevated cholesterol, or that the patient drinks or eats too much, the physician can only urge, cajole, admonish, or refer the patient to a nutritionist or counselor.

Physicians don't usually engage in teaching patients how to modify their life-styles, how to *prevent* disease. Rarely do they have the time or the skills. This issue is the key to a new style of medical practice that's needed today, and is probably the reason you bought this book.

Up until recently—say, the past twenty years or so—people were encouraged to see doctors for simple reasons: they had developed either a symptom or a signal that something was wrong—something ached, or, in some cases, something in the body was working poorly, or not at all. Poor health was thought by most people to be simply the result of bad luck. When someone died suddenly, physicians could often only guess as to the cause. But since World War II, a great deal of research attention has been paid to what shortens people's lives: what causes illnesses to appear and what can be done in terms of day-to-day living to *prevent* them, not simply cure them.

One of these studies, which became known as the Framingham Study, examined people in that Massachusetts town beginning in 1947. After twenty years, scientists concluded that elevated blood pressure, high blood cholesterol or blood sugar levels, and life-style-linked habits such as cigarette smoking tremendously increased the likelihood that someone would have a premature heart attack or stroke.

The Framingham Study generated data that became the standard by which cardiovascular risk is now estimated throughout the world. In fact, a term we will use frequently in this book—*risk factor*, a measurement of the magnitude of your potential to get sick—was developed by the insurance industry when it realized that data from studies like this could help identify people who might die prematurely and could therefore affect profits.

Subsequent studies have shown that many other illnesses—some cancers, some complications of pregnancy and accidents, in fact, some thirty-plus diseases—each have their own antecedent characteristics or identifiable risk factors. And many risk factors are linked directly to life-style. If these can be eliminated or even just reduced, the chances of disease developing are also reduced. It sounds simple and it *is* simple.

But in order to practice good health behavior successfully and to stay out of the doctor's office as much as possible, you must get to know your exact health risks at various stages of your life. Once you understand these risks clearly, you can then learn the skills required to beat the odds.

MAKING THIS BOOK WORK FOR YOU

Risk estimation, the basis for *Beat the Odds*, is a very new scientific tool that combines the use of computers and statistics, self-health-care knowledge, and your personal occupational, social, and medical history along with medical histories of your peers.

Your personal health risks can be estimated by matching information about yourself against computerized data available for the rest of the population. Data bases that give an average profile of the entire population are compared by the computer with your personal profile. The results let you see which of several hundred specific characteristics you match, and which you don't.

Beat the Odds is the world's first personally interactive health book, because it provides you with a way to learn your *exact* health risks: just fill out the enclosed *Beat the Odds Health Questionnaire* and mail it to the General Health Inc. health risk appraisal program for a complete computerized analysis.

When we decided to create a book based on mainstream medical techniques for reducing health risks, we knew that the only way to do this was to find some method of letting the reader learn his or her own specific risks. We contacted many companies who specialize in this type of computerized evaluation for major corporations, to help them plan employee health-care programs. The leader in the field was General Health Inc. located in Washington, D.C.

Our research into risk-appraisal technology helped us to understand that the data base used and the methodology on which the appraisal is based are critical when personal health risks are assessed. We chose General Health's health risk appraisal program for *Beat the Odds* quite simply because it utilizes the finest, most up-to-date data base in existence today. General Health Inc. (GHI) is internationally recognized for its technical excellence in health-management products and services. Its qualified staff includes physicians, epidemiologists, biostatisticians, psychologists, software designers, program analysts, and communications specialists in offices all over the country. GHI's skills are employed by such major corporations as IBM and Blue Cross/Blue Shield.

WHAT IS "HEALTH RISK APPRAISAL"?

On the opening pages of this book you will find simple, thorough instructions for completion of the initial *Beat the Odds Health Questionnaire,* which you must fill out in order to get the ball rolling. When you've completed this task, slip the *BTO Questionnaire* into the enclosed envelope along with the required seven-dollar fee, and send it off—no postage required—to GHI.

You will receive in the mail a complete, twelve-page *Beat the Odds Health Profile,* which will give you very specific information about your health risks. The *BTO Profile* will also direct you to those parts of this book that are particularly relevant as far as helping you personally to beat the odds.

As you fill out the *BTO Questionnaire,* you'll answer queries about your medical history, physical data, and personal life-style habits. *Please note that you are asked some very specific questions about cholesterol levels, blood pressure levels, etcetera. (Questions 1.07 to 1.14) This information will help us get a more accurate picture of your health, so if you don't know the answers, ask your doctor. Although we can process your questionnaire without this data, your results will be more complete if you can obtain this information. If you've never had these tests done, ask your doctor to arrange for them.*

GHI's computers analyze your data, comparing your responses with a huge data base of information and statistics to produce your own individual *Beat the Odds Health Profile,* reporting on your chances of becoming ill or even possibly dying from specific diseases.

While this may sound complicated, the premise behind it is simple. The *BTO Profile,* using computer technology developed by GHI, synthesizes and analyzes a great deal of health information drawn from hundreds of studies on the health of millions of Americans. Since the computer automatically reads and reports to *you,* make sure you fill out the *BTO Questionnaire* as accurately and completely as possible. If you leave any responses blank, the *BTO Profile* results may not reflect all of your personal characteristics.

These characteristics (the so-called risk indicators) might be your blood pressure levels, the amount of exercise you do compared with that of the rest of the population of your age, or your cholesterol levels. The information in GHI's data base tells us whether the level of your blood pressure or your current exercise program has any particular health consequences. For example, is your pressure too high or your exercise program inadequate?

Once you have an idea of what your various risk indicators are, you'll also want to know just how much you are at risk—what the magnitude of your health risk is. When your risk indicators are compared to others of your age, sex, race, etcetera, you will know if your risk factors constitute a serious problem or not.

These risk factors are considered measures of your specific potential health problems. If your risk factors are similar to the average for your age, sex, race, etcetera, then your estimated risk factor will be about average. Some risk factors—such as age, sex, race, and family history—are obviously unchangeable. But others—blood pressure levels, sugar intake, weight, physical activity, to cite a few—can be changed.

If you have several risk factors of a greater magnitude than the average, you can expect to have more serious health problems than the rest of the population, unless you take steps to modify your lifestyle and lower those risks.

An analysis of your risk factors will be contained in your own *Beat the Odds Health Profile*. *Remember, it is a statement of statistical probability, not a specific diagnosis.*

The *BTO Profile* is your own tool for initiating change. But where do you learn *how* to change behavior? This is one of the questions we discuss and answer in this book. We will show you how to combine the risk factor identification you receive in your *BTO Profile* with an education in how to change behavior that puts you at risk. *Beat the Odds* first tells you your health risks, then gives you reasonable strategies for appropriate behavioral change.

You should use this book over and over again, referring back to it whenever you lose your way. Write in the margins! Dog-ear the pages! This book is your own guide to reducing health risks. Use it and beat the odds against you for premature illness and death.

Now fill out the *BTO Questionnaire*, mail it to GHI, and read on to find out how to use this book and your *BTO Profile*.

HOW TO USE THIS BOOK

Finding out about your own health risks and correcting them is not designed to be a difficult task. It should not create anxiety and fear; rather, it should be a reassuring experience. From your *Beat the Odds Health Profile*, you'll find out which parts of your life are lived properly and which parts you can change to beat the odds.

Chapters One through Twelve in this book are designed to give you strategies on how to reduce risks to safe levels. You begin by following the instructions in your *BTO Profile*. But before you do, here's some information on how to use that profile.

If you have taken the time to fill out the *BTO Questionnaire*, you're probably eager to receive your *BTO Profile* and learn more about your personal health risks and how to improve them. And once you receive the *BTO Profile*, you may be interested in learning just how your risks are calculated.

EXAMINING YOUR BTO PROFILE

Now, take a look at your *BTO Profile* results.

The inside cover tells you what you can expect to learn from your *BTO Profile*—what it does, and does not, do. Keep in mind that while the *BTO Profile* is an excellent guide to your personal health risks and how to improve them, it, like this book, is not meant to be a substitute for your regular or other needed visits to a doctor.

Our premise throughout this book is that beating the odds requires information about your health risks, strategies for a healthy life-style, and partnership with a physician who can address your problems as an individual.

Pages 2 to 5 and pages 8 to 11 of the *BTO Profile* talk about risk areas—those areas of your everyday life-style that have a major impact on your health. One page side of the *BTO Profile* offers you a thumbnail sketch of what each risk area is, how it affects your health, and why it's so important.

WHAT THE RISK AREA MEANS TO YOU

On the opposite page side of the *BTO Profile*, you'll see how that particular risk area affects your own personal health. These pages focus on the four leading causes of death: heart attack, stroke, motor vehicle accidents, and cancer.

In each case, you will see your personal health risk, how that risk compares to that of others your age, and, finally, how much you could reduce your health risks if all of your risk factors were at ideal levels.

Perhaps some of your risk factors fall within the average range.

Don't think that means you are as healthy as you could possibly be, and that you don't have to give that risk area any further thought. "Average" does not necessarily mean "healthy." Even if your risk factor is average or better, there still may be room for improvement. *The "average" American has a risk of heart attack many times greater than other populations in the world.*

On the other hand, don't be alarmed or discouraged if your risk factors are higher than you had expected. Remember, by making conscious changes in your daily behavior, you have the ability to affect significantly many of your risk factor levels.

HOW DO YOU KNOW WHAT SPECIFIC CHANGES TO MAKE?

That's easy. Look at the bottom of each personal risk level page, where you are directed to relevant pages in this book. There you will learn specific *strategies* for improving your health—practical suggestions you and your family can follow to live longer, healthier lives.

For instance, pages 8 and 9 of your *BTO Profile* might tell you that by losing weight you can reduce your risk of heart attack and stroke, adding several years to your life span. At the bottom of the weight section on page 8, you will see which chapters in *Beat the Odds* deal with losing weight. In those chapters you'll learn a wealth of information about such things as food values, the way to make permanent dietary changes to reduce cholesterol intake, and the difference between "dieting" and having a proper diet.

Perhaps your *BTO Profile* tells you that there are a number of life-style changes you need to make. Don't feel you have to make several major changes overnight or all at once. Such expectations are unrealistic and will likely set you up for potential failure. Instead, think about making small changes, taking small steps, one at a time. Also, you may be wondering which aspects of your life-style are *most* important to change. Turn to page 12 of your *BTO Profile*, where you'll find the different behaviors ranked in order of their impact on your health.

No one ever said that changing long-time habits is easy. But page 10 of your *BTO Profile* will give you a few quick tips on ways to make your job less difficult.

One important thing to keep in mind is repeated several times in this book: *Behavior change is far less difficult if you feel you're not in it alone*. It's tough to change your poor diet when the person across the dinner table is feasting on a chocolate triple-layer cake, and, conversely, it's easier to dine on a healthy salad when everyone else at the table is eating it, too. So try to make these changes in your health a family affair. Get your family involved in using this book, too.

If you'd like to get *Beat the Odds Health Profiles* for family members or friends, so that they can use the guidance in *Beat the Odds*, simply write to General Health Inc., 3299 K Street, N.W., Washington, D.C. 20007, or call GHI at (800) 424-2775, during East Coast business hours; they will send you additional copies of the *Beat the Odds Health Questionnaire*. Enclose $7 for each additional questionnaire.

How We Will Beat the Odds in the Future

WHY WE WROTE THIS BOOK

Several years ago, my colleagues and I at the Brigham and Women's Hospital in Boston wrote a self-help workbook on cardiac risk reduction, to be used by patients in our Healthstyle program. We created the workbook because we recognized that, despite our own knowledge about health risks and our feeling that a person can become a "successful patient" through education, we needed to teach risk-reduction techniques to our patients, too. So this book contains both information about disease and "how to" information about changing behavior.

Our research at that time showed me that if I told somebody simply to "lose weight," the patient was likely to drop out of my care. I was trying to treat people with high blood pressure, maturity-onset diabetes, or hyperlipidemia (high cholesterol levels), yet I was not able to do anything about their weight—a major risk factor—because of a Catch-22 contradiction. If I told them initially to do something about their weight, they would drop out of care; if I didn't tell them to do something beside take medication, I was neglecting my responsibility.

So I began using a workbook to help people learn about their health and learn strategies for change. I was surprised at the number of people who began to pay attention. Once they got interested in changing their diets, losing weight, or quitting smoking, they would be inspired to do it on their own or would respond to recommended programs outside the office.

Not only was I surprised at the success of the Healthstyle workbook, but I was impressed by how many people, when given tangible information, would take the book home, read it, and use it. Their wives or husbands would read it, too, and they would also help in making changes. Finally I was convinced that a doctor could teach health and the practice of health while still maintaining the traditional role and services that people expected. And my experience with The Silver Fox, which I described earlier, confirmed my feeling about reaching people with information.

But my practice is limited to the Greater Boston area and my time is spread between Healthstyle and the Harvard Medical School. How could anyone take advantage of the Healthstyle education process, become a responsible medical consumer, and still maintain an interactive relationship with a doctor that is so vital to improving health risks?

One way was to incorporate General Health Inc.'s health risk appraisal technology with a cogent, behaviorally correct set of instructions in a book like this. Although we couldn't incorporate every single principle of education, we could cover the ones that really count. We could help a person, through identification of health risks, to deal with situations he or she is commonly faced with in the doctor's office. We could help a patient focus on things that the doctor has not clearly explained.

Beat the Odds is intended to combine a way to identify your own individual health risks with a way to change your specific health-related behaviors. The difference between this approach and all others is we do not set up punitive lists of do's and don'ts. Instead, solutions are given in which people really have enough latitude to develop some of their own strategies.

This book is not to be looked at as a substitute for the doctor/patient interaction. (If information in this book conflicts with your physician's views, discuss these conflicts directly.) My view is that today a physician should be (but is not always) the conduit through which health information should flow and through which feedback is obtained. Reinforcement and monitoring by a doctor is still one of the most important aspects of preventive health care. It's vital that you have a physician who knows you. For example, if you are my patient, and you call me up at four in the afternoon and say, "I'm having chest pain," then I can call upon my records and recollections to help integrate what I know about you to explain that chest pain.

We've written this book, partially, because we feel the roles of physician and patient *must* change as risk reduction becomes a more important part of medical care in the 1980s. And we've written this book to spread our knowledge of successful methods of risk reduction in the context of the traditional roles that doctors and patients will continue to play.

OUR MEDICAL RISK-REDUCTION SYSTEM IS DEVELOPING

Despite continual publicity about health risks in the daily press, the idea that personal risk factors can be controlled is a relatively new concept in medical practice. In fact, there is so much publicity about health risks that almost no one understands what the subject is all about. For example, we are continually confusing the *nature* of health risks and the *significance* of certain health risks—flu epidemics are an example—to the general population.

There is also a difference between *personal* health risk factors and overall *public* health risks in a specific situation. Personal and public health hazards may be intertwined, but your actual control over the two may be vastly different.

What kinds of public health risks do we hear about most today? For one thing, we *always* hear about airplane crashes and drug scares like the Tylenol poisonings. Generally we read about "disaster" in regard to personal safety. When the Union Carbide tragedy in Bhopal, India, occurred, we were treated to daily doses of the "potential threat" from chemical accidents. In reality, very few of us are threatened by chemical plant accidents. But we react to these front-page stories with increased fear of flying or a temporary reluctance to use a product that had previously always been effective.

Why? According to research carried out by Dr. John Urquhart and Dr. Klaus Heilmann, presented in their book *Risk Watch* (Facts on File, 1984), "The reports we receive in the news media of [health risk] catastrophes and other untoward events are victim-oriented, as in 'Fourteen Die of Mystery Disease.'"

They point out that most reports of disasters don't tell us "how many people altogether were in danger, how many may have gotten sick and recovered, how many never got sick, and so on." Fourteen people may have died out of 100 million potential victims, making the odds 14:100,000,000 that the disease will affect you, but the impact of how it's reported is out of proportion to the threat.

Victim-oriented reporting, especially in the area of health risks, "tends to leave us with free-floating anxiety and dread about such things as—in no particular order—the bomb, the next earthquake, air pollution, car crashes, jet crashes, lead poisoning, toxic shock syndrome, deformed babies, chemical plant explosions, carcinogens in food, asbestos in drinking water, cancer risk of X rays, passive smoking, mercury and seafoods, dioxin, and so on," Urquhart and Heilmann say.

What has happened to our society is that we tend to look at risks from the point of view of how many *were* injured or affected rather than those who *weren't*. To combat this distortion, a number of degree-of-safety scales have been devised to put risk in perspective. We know, using these scales, that despite the massive publicity that occurs when a plane goes down, air travel is actually very safe.

We also know, according to established measures, that cigarette smoking is far more dangerous to us than drowning due to a flood or a tornado. Still, floods and similar disasters receive much more publicity than the hundreds who die each day from the effects of tobacco.

By learning about "actual" risks, our society can put the emphasis on prevention—where it really belongs. And each person can also do

Risk of Flying

YEAR	NUMBER OF VICTIMS	NUMBER OF PASSENGERS
1960	499	62,000,000
1965	261	103,000,000
1970	146	169,000,000
1974	467	208,000,000
1975	124	205,000,000
1976	45	223,000,000
1977	655	240,000,000
1978	163	275,000,000
1979	353	317,000,000

Adapted from *Risk Watch,* by John Urquhart, M.D., and Klaus Heilmann, M.D. (New York: Facts on File, 1984).

Relative Risks—Various Hazards and Their Per-Year Risk of Death

RISK	1 DEATH PER YEAR PER:
Cigarette smoking	600 (smokers)
Motorcycles	1,000 (passengers)
Automobiles	6,000 (passengers)
Oral contraceptives	23,000 (users, ages 25–34)
Pedestrians	26,000
Cycling	88,000
Tornadoes	450,000
Lightning	1,900,000
Bee stings	5,500,000
Hit by falling airplanes	10,000,000
Drowning due to flooded dikes (Netherlands)	10,000,000

Adapted from *Risk Watch,* by John Urquhart, M.D., and Klaus Heilmann, M.D. (New York: Facts on File, 1984).

the same. In addition, we can learn that a "risk" is not a "cause." For example, a cigarette puts you at risk for lung cancer, while a plane crash may be the actual "cause" of your death.

As the discipline of epidemiology has developed, we have learned how to measure risks, but we have not really learned how to put them in perspective—to incorporate them into our lives. There are several reasons besides "victim-oriented reporting." First, statistical methods are a relatively new way of looking at things, and, second, it is not always easy to obtain accurate data. There are laws protecting certain types of personal records, so it often takes many years for a risk factor to become evident. People also tend to be suspicious of "scientific data." Plus, we tend to balance a potential risk—such as driving a car—with a potential benefit—convenience—despite the low degree of safety that activity may imply.

We have also seen that as society becomes more aware of the perspective in which health risks should be placed, we tend to make risk:benefit decisions personally. We decide when and if we are going to drive a car, smoke cigarettes, or fly in a plane. We decide if we are going to live in a polluted city or the pristine countryside for personal reasons. We are generally aware of the "big risks" when we make these decisions, but we assume someone else—the government or the health professionals—will protect us. We think "they" would not let us buy cigarettes if they were *that* bad for us. We have not, until recently, spent much time focusing on how we can identify and change our own personal health risks.

Why has it taken so long for us to determine that we can reduce health risks by ourselves? One of the reasons lies in the historical development of the concept of risk reduction.

A BRIEF HISTORY OF HEALTH RISKS

When Edward Jenner first successfully inoculated the English population against smallpox, he became the "godfather of preventive medicine." Interestingly, although Jenner's vaccine was first used in 1792, it was not until 1979 that the World Health Organization declared smallpox eradicated. Concepts like vaccination were actually resisted for many decades. It was felt that scientists who advocated such measures were interfering with the "natural order" of life. Further, none of these and other similar procedures were without side effects or risk, and they required brave scientists to recommend them.

Since it was often a very costly and complicated procedure to lower certain health risks, many earlier generations did not feel it was worth it to do so. In addition, in the past, as today, there were bureaucrats and politicians who kept information from the public for their own reasons. Urquhart and Heilmann point out that the problems faced by Jenner and his colleagues were not all that different from those faced by the U.S. Public Health Service when it declared that the "swine flu" epidemic of the late 1970s could rival the great influenza epidemic of 1918. When it became known that the flu vaccine had a "potential" side effect, the program was abruptly dropped, and most of the officials involved lost their jobs.

During the growth of this country, from colonial times to the early twentieth century, vaccination and other general public health measures, such as sewer drainage or draining swamps to eliminate malaria, were our only efforts at controlling health risks.

Personal risk reduction also was not considered an important task because as late as the 1930s or 1940s, most diseases were still thought to occur randomly. That is, people believed they occurred as a measure of some sort of religious shortcoming, as a failure of good luck, or some other reason.

By looking at high blood pressure and cigarette smoking as important—yet personal—public health risks, we can see just how long it took for the idea of personal health risks to alter our consciousness.

The adverse effects of high blood pressure were first reported in

1923. The potential dangers of smoking were first noted about 1940 in the medical literature.

By the late thirties and early forties, some physician-scientists with "primitive tools" were sure that high blood pressure and cigarette smoking were "bad" for people. As early as 1940, Gerald Burch at the Ochsner clinic in New Orleans began writing about the health hazards of cigarette smoking. As epidemiology came into its own in the 1950s, we began to see hard evidence that smokers were fifteen times more likely to develop lung cancer than nonsmokers. We also learned from long-term studies of smokers that they faced other health hazards, such as cardiovascular disease. Finally, in 1963, the Surgeon General of the United States presented his classic report on the potential health hazards associated with smoking. Cigarettes, we discovered, were the single greatest "voluntary" health hazard we faced.

Smoking again came under fire as a personal health risk when the Build and Blood Pressure Study of 1939 began showing evidence that cigarette smoking and high blood pressure were linked health hazards that contributed to heart attack and stroke. Very soon after that, insurance companies started recording blood pressure and smoking habits as part of their physical exams.

Most people don't remember that blood pressure recording didn't start until the turn of the century. In fact, it was not until 1923 that the Mayo Clinic published a study about a health hazard they called "malignant hypertension." By 1929, the original patients studied in 1923 had all died, and this confirmed that some form of hypertension was truly a malignant process. And, like smoking, we began to see that high blood pressure posed public health problems, that it was a risk both to the general population and to each of us as individuals.

By 1950, it was suspected that even lower levels of high blood pressure—asymptomatic—also caused people to die early of strokes and heart failure. We finally began to get hard evidence that with high blood pressure levels, even though you are young and have no symptoms and feel well, you could have a condition likely to shorten your life.

As far as cigarettes were concerned, as early as the forties and fifties, more people began to smoke, despite some two thousand medical reports at that time that cigarette smoking was a health hazard. In fact, as the tobacco industry grew, smoking became something more than a habit—it became "chic."

In the late 1950s, for the first time, people finally began to believe that personal risk factors were as serious—if not more serious—than the symptoms of disease they already had. Yet we still did not embrace the idea that we could do much about this problem, because effective treatment tools were not available then. For example, the early drugs used for control of high blood pressure had serious and potentially fatal side effects. Not until the late 1950s did we start to find medications whose side effects were not as bad as the potential diseases they were supposed to cure.

But more and more health officials were concerned, and in the early 1940s, beginning with the Framingham Study, it was decided to do several long-term population studies that would categorically determine just how widespread these risk factor problems really were and what could be done about them.

Even as these studies were conducted, overall public health was improving, as demonstrated by our lengthening life span. Antibiotic drugs were in widespread use now, and sanitary conditions were the norm, rather than the exception. The first half of the twentieth century had been the era of penicillin and other medical breakthroughs that improved public health. It seemed possible that the second half could be an era of improved overall personal health.

As we mentioned, the information generated by these studies gradually became accepted because the insurance industry utilized the data to determine how risk factors affected life and insurance health premiums. Thus it was economics that spurred our understanding and embrace of personal health risk reduction.

When we entered the golden age of pharmaceuticals in the 1940s, along with better general health care, we also became more aware of risk reduction. Wonder drugs, along with better surgical techniques and diagnostic tools, allowed us to live long enough to develop heart disease or stroke, which are now understood as diseases whose crippling or fatal symptoms take years to develop. During this time we also looked at "treatment-related risks," to gauge the side effects: benefit ratio of drugs.

As far as personal risk reduction goes, the first great breakthrough in medicine was the advent of routine blood pressure screening. Today, almost everyone has blood pressure examinations on a regular basis, on the job or in a variety of other settings.

In my opinion, the ensuing reduction in stroke and heart disease over the last twenty years ranks the blood pressure exam in the same league as the discovery of penicillin, so far as personal health is concerned. Recognizing that people can identify and then control their own risk factors with regular blood pressure readings is as significant as anything else medicine has done in this century. It's interesting to note, also, that the awareness and treatment of high blood pressure has been the result of efforts of many people, including government agencies, volunteer agencies such as the American Heart Association, the pharmaceutical industry, health educators, nurses, and physicians.

We later became aware and now really believe that people's life-styles can adversely affect their health—that, just as with high blood pressure levels, they can have asymptomatic conditions that predict premature morbidity and mortality. This belief will cause—indeed, is causing—a permanent transformation in the way medicine is practiced. Most likely, doctors and patients will never be the same. Risk reduction, we hope, will forever be a part of the "practice of health" in this country.

REDEFINING ROLES IN MEDICAL PRACTICE

Today, we are first beginning to see the impact of the control of personal risk factors as a significant part of a physician's medical practice. But physicians lag behind industry and the medical consumer movement, both of which have already embraced personal risk reduction. The life insurance companies are now educating people about health risks because it's in their best economic interests to have healthier clients.

The communicators—journalists, teachers, even the alternative medicine advocates—are also educating people. And they are passing the physician on the highway. Why has this happened, in view of the fact that, historically, the medical profession has been in the forefront of prevention as a general public health measure?

Mostly because we as physicians were and are primarily trained to be *treaters* of disease rather than *preventers* of illness. Doctors don't as a rule talk about practicing good health behavior because they spend most of their training learning how to cure disease. Interns and residents are hospital-based; they are very good at treating the end stages of prevention—actually, often the failures of prevention.

Few medical schools place training in preventive medicine high on their list of priorities. High-tech medicine and computer-oriented treatments and research are more attractive to medical students, whose undergraduate education has been steeped in science, not the humanities.

Despite the fact that we have finally changed the public's attitude about health risks through education, we are now only beginning to train doctors to help reduce risks in the other type of patient we see—the type classified as "ambulatory well."

The ambulatory well—defined as people who show up in a doctor's office for treatment of minor aches and pains, colds, and the flu—have always been a large part of the family doctor's practice. You used to go to a doctor once a year for a checkup. The doctor would take your blood pressure and it might be a little high. You might be overweight, you might smoke, but the general message the doctor gave you was "You are fine. You seem well, I didn't see a cancer on your X ray. You don't have an enlarged liver." But then you may have walked out of the doctor's office and dropped dead in the street of a heart attack. So apparently you were not all right, just "ambulatory well."

Because this happened so frequently, we as physicians now earnestly started to consider the issue of prevention. We began to debate among ourselves on how to change current practice, or, if an attempt should even be made to make people understand and embrace the idea of risk reduction.

There was no question among us that you should have all kinds of diagnostic tests done routinely. But most doctors weren't and aren't geared up to monitor their patients' test requirements. For this they would need statistical printouts that would chart the progress of each individual patient. In the standard practice in this country, the physician sees between three and five thousand patients a year. Thus it's virtually impossible for a doctor to look at a patient's chart and say, "This man last had a chest X ray at forty years and one should be repeated on January fifth. He last had his sigmoidoscopy seven years ago and one should be repeated on December twelfth." Only a statistical workup could provide this information readily.

Most doctors contend that the economy can't bear that much monitoring and testing, but that's not really why this type of medicine is not routinely practiced in this country. It is not so much that the economy can't bear it, but that patients are conditioned to rely too much on the doctor to make these decisions.

What we should be saying is, it is time for people to participate more actively in the monitoring of their own health once doctors have identified their personal risk factors.

"Doctor," each person should be saying, "why haven't I had a stress test? Should I have a barium enema and sigmoidoscopy? Should I get a flu shot? Why have I not been given x, y, and z?"

The doctor/patient encounter is often one in which the patient doesn't want to be in the doctor's office any longer than he has to and the doctor wants to go on to the next patient as quickly as possible. For this and other reasons, our medical system has encouraged and enabled people other than physicians to become teachers of health skills. We are at the start of a process that will ultimately include the physician in part of the teaching of health skills, so that doctors will not just be participants in a series of symptom/disease curing encounters.

There is no question that American physicians excel at treating disease. Nowhere in the world, and nowhere in the history of mankind, have so many resources been marshaled to treat disease as well as it is treated now in this country. We understand more, and have more diagnostic tools. It is amazing to see how rapidly the treatment of disease has progressed.

We have reached the point now where it is getting harder and harder to die. Doctors are so good at keeping you alive that they can put a plastic heart in your chest and keep you alive until a heart transplant is available. They can provide you with transplants of your liver, your kidneys, your corneas, your lungs, and quite a few other parts. In other words, death can be postponed almost indefinitely. We have made great progress in treating cancer, and this scientific inquiry in medicine *must* be encouraged. . . .

. . . *But we have missed the point, both as physicians and as patients.* For all of us, our principal mission together should be to postpone the premature appearance of those illnesses that are preventable by identifying risk factors and helping to reduce them. This is the new task for the physician and the patient in the 1980s.

BECOMING A PATIENT—THE ULTIMATE CONSUMER

As we take on our new jobs—both of us—there will emerge physicians more adept at teaching risk reduction and patients less afraid to take responsibility for and participate in their own care. This will be accomplished by both M.D. and patient adopting different roles than they have traditionally played. The major difference for patients is that they will have to participate more—to learn about illness and prevention, to learn strategies for change. The patient will become less of a passive participant, and the physician will have become more of a health educator.

Suppose you go to the doctor for a checkup. The doctor examines you and says your blood pressure is high. But you have no symptoms. The traditional clues, such as pain and dysfunction, are not there. So you're not convinced that there is anything wrong with you, certainly not if you compare yourself, let's say, to someone with a broken leg.

But still, the doctor says, "Your blood pressure is 160 over 100, and you need to make certain changes in your life." Then the doctor recites a long list of changes, such as these:

- You need to eliminate salt from your diet.
- You need to exercise.
- You need to lose weight and learn to relax.
- Perhaps you could supplement your diet with certain minerals, such as potassium or calcium.

The list goes on: take pills, buy a home monitor, etcetera. You walk out of the doctor's office and say, "Gee, I feel okay, but this is an enormous shopping list of things to do. I understand what he said to me, but this is a long list of changes."

What you really feel, unlike the patient with the broken leg, is that the benefits—which are not immediate—are not worth the high cost of giving up much of your life-style.

I won't feel better or look better, you think. There are no immediate payoffs, like relief of pain or suffering, and the cost to my time and my life-style is enormous. Few people at age 35 with asymptomatic high blood pressure can project themselves into a hospital bed with a heart attack at age 55.

In many cases—perhaps 50 percent—patients may not even believe they have a problem. All their denial mechanisms come into play, and they drop out of care.

Why does this happen so often?

Because virtually *all* risk-reduction processes deal with asymptomatic situations.

If a patient has hypertension so out of control that it causes headaches, and if the medication you give the patient makes the headaches go away, then you have not only reduced risk, you have also relieved a symptom. This has a built-in reinforcement that will keep the patient coming back.

What Do We Mean by Health?

Here is the only really relevant definition: *Health is something that most people have and never give any thought to until they lose it.*

This definition, when understood in the context of risk reduction, can help you stay on the fast track without killing yourself. But to change your belief system—or your disbelief system—there has to be a process called internalization.

You have to say, "I don't want to wind up like the guy they carried out of the board meeting." And you have to mean it.

With this type of redefinition, many people will immediately reset their sights and make some life-style changes, adjusting their health practices.

But in most cases of hypertension and other conditions that do not affect a person's ability to function, treatment makes people feel no better.

That's why another important aspect of becoming a patient in the 1980s, as you learn how to beat the odds, is to accept a different explanation of what "being healthy" really means.

DEVELOPING HEALTH SKILLS WON'T BE EASY

In order to prevent illness and make the process of becoming a patient easier, both doctors and patients need to develop skills that help them practice preventive medicine—*health skills.*

To practice these skills—developing a healthy diet, creating an exercise program, working on stress and weight-reduction strategies—people need to learn new methods of operation. This isn't simple. For example, if I told you to go out and learn to play tennis, you would have to take lessons, perhaps even join a club. You would have to find a teacher and somebody to practice with as you build your skill. A learning process has to take place.

When you take a college course, the teacher says, "Here is the material you should read tonight." You go home and read it, and the next day you go to class and discuss it with the teacher. You correct any misunderstandings you have, and then at the end of the week, you have a quiz to reinforce your knowledge of the information. And three months later, when the final exam comes along, you have yet another test to make sure that this subject has become a permanent or integrated part of your knowledge.

The college course embodies sound educational principles, as do the tennis lessons. You are required to be motivated, to learn the material, and to reinforce your knowledge with practice. Only after following this specific method will the information or the skill be yours.

How can a doctor in his office today reproduce those principles of education?

As the practice of medicine is currently structured, a visit to a doctor's office is not set up as a learning situation. Your doctor can identify your health risks and even attempt to give you motivation to want change. But the doctor visit is not structured—economically, time-wise, or even training-wise—to give you the kinds of skills you have to develop to learn about health.

During an extensive three-year patient-compliance research program that I directed in the late 1970s, I came in contact with two educators, Dr. Patricia McArdle and Dr. Marion Field Fass. As we carried out the work, I was introduced daily to new principles of education and how they applied to the physician/patient encounter. I marveled at these new discoveries, and as I discussed them each night with my wife, who is also an educator, she would smile and nod her head, saying, "Sure—Ed. Psych. 101." What teachers learn as a basic skill early in their training, physicians also need to know. But they have usually never even heard about such things.

Another barrier to using the doctor visit as a learning process is that it does not provide a good atmosphere for teaching; there is too much anxiety around going to the doctor for it to serve as an effective situation for information transfer. And, you don't go to the doctor expecting to *learn*—you go to be cured or diagnosed. All too often, the expectation of a person going to a doctor is that the doctor will "do something."

Let's suppose that a patient has come to me for treatment of an annoying cough. I do a complete physical exam, and the only thing I find wrong after an extensive evaluation is that the patient smokes too much and has a little bit of bronchitis.

I bring the patient back a week later, sit down, and say, "Let's talk about smoking and how to change smoking behavior." I may even spend forty-five minutes talking about how to stop smoking successfully.

No prescription is given, no medicine, nothing. The patient walks away. All too often—unlike The Silver Fox—the patient will say, "That doctor didn't *do* anything for me. All I got was a lecture about smoking." A basic problem—as doctors try to redefine their roles so they can help people reduce risks—is that people expect "something for their money," like a shot, or a pill, or a treatment. They want some *thing*.

This problem of patient expectations is certainly one of the reasons that diagnostic studies are overused. That a "complete" physical exam should include a urine analysis and EKG, whether called for or not, is really to make patients think they are getting a "complete" physical exam (some *thing* for their money). It may be that the smoking is the primary health issue, or the patient's 30-pounds-overweight prediabetic state is the issue, but the patient isn't there for a lecture.

After this "complete" exam, many doctors send the patient a letter saying, basically:

"You are 30 pounds overweight and you need to lose weight to correct your possible diabetes or cholesterol problems. I'll see you next year."

In the interval the patient has a heart attack and asks, What the hell happened?

What happened was the physician was trapped—caught between what he knows is the way to practice risk reduction and the expectations of the American patient. He's caught between his extraordinary skills as a treater of disease and the patient-expectation system that keeps him from teaching health skills.

Are the Times Finally Changing?

I am hopeful that all other physicians in this country will begin to teach their patients about health risk reduction. It continues to amaze me that more isn't being done as medicine becomes more cost-conscious. Moreover, the population seems to want this information. Every time I get on an airplane now and read the airline magazines, I see an article on "10 Ways to Fix Tofu" or fifteen different articles on stress reduction in every possible environment.

When corporation executives go out for business lunches now, they eat salads and drink soda water with a twist of lime. The macho image is changing. A business lunch of steak and potatoes and three martinis is not as common as it once was. In fact, a recent story in *Newsweek* was called "Let's *Not* Have Lunch," and confirmed this "fitness trend."

More people will become much more aware of the importance of risk reduction as society embraces it as an economic necessity. But what we still lack is more in-depth understanding. We need something else from our "teacher–doctors" to understand how to become patients and really begin to change.

For example, a doctor will say to a patient: "Your cholesterol is a little high; it is 275 and it should be 220."

What does that mean to me? the patient should ask.

What is the *risk* of having a cholesterol level of 275 compared to having one of 220? Most physicians are not really equipped to answer that question, yet it means that the person with the higher number has a three times greater risk of heart disease.

Most doctors also don't talk in terms of *multiple risks.*

For example, what happens if your blood pressure is mildly elevated, say, 140 over 95, and your cholesterol level is 300? What is the difference between having that kind of risk profile and having your cholesterol at 200 with the same blood pressure?

The truth is, there is no ready answer, like "You'll die in six years if you don't change." But there are ways to express these situations in terms of "risk" or "odds"—just take a look at your *Beat the Odds Health Profile.* We have a receptive public but too few tools to serve them with.

Another barrier to helping patients understand risk factors is that lowering cholesterol through regular monitoring has not until recently been a priority. Certainly, without the latest studies clearly showing that diet and drug therapy lower cholesterol levels and cardiovascular risk—our greatest threat—we'd still be far behind the consumer advocates with ammunition to convince people to lower consumption of saturated fats. Remember that even physicians whose teaching skills are superb and whose awareness of risk factors is keen are still limited in what they can do. Physicians are held accountable in different ways from those applied to the popular press or a consumer critic. Doctors must back up what they say with hard scientific evidence or else they are at risk for suit.

Hopefully, what will happen as far as learning about our risks from cholesterol is that there will be a National High Cholesterol Education Program analogous to the National High Blood Pressure Education Program, which had such a major impact on our understanding of hypertension.

DO CHANGING DIETS REFLECT OUR "RISK AWARENESS QUOTIENT"?

Diet is really a very major determinant of health in ways we do and do not understand. This is why we dwell on different aspects of *diet,* not *dieting,* in Chapters Six and Twelve. While we do have some data on the relationship of diet to cardiovascular disease, in the coming years we hope to learn much more about diet's relationship to cancer, bone disease, and other health problems.

The way we eat now and the way our diet is changing is a good indicator of the way Americans will approach risk reduction to beat the odds, once properly instructed. Thus the subject bears a little closer inspection.

We know there is nothing inherently "wrong" with eating eggs and there is nothing "wrong" with eating fried foods. There is nothing wrong with eating fat-laden French cuisine either. What *is* wrong is that some of us eat too much of those kinds of food. For many people, fat has become a staple of their diet rather than an exception to it. What you and I used to eat for Sunday dinner once a week has become a seven-day-a-week event. Ice cream used to be an occasional treat; now, with home freezers, ice cream is available all the time. That is why the American public as a whole has developed risk factors related to diet.

Americans essentially eat less now than they did at the turn of the century. But more of us are overweight. It is estimated that only about 10 percent of the population was overweight around the turn of the century; now 30 percent of us are overweight, while eating less.

What has happened over the ensuing eighty years is that fewer people earn their livelihood with physical labor. For the first time in history, more of us now work in information processing than in the production of goods. More of us sit down to work than tote barges and lift bales.

Until the turn of the century, nobody in the country was concerned with nutritional excess. Rather, we were concerned that there was too little food. Malnutrition was a worldwide problem and continues to be for the vast majority of the world. Excessive nourishment is unique to a minority of the world's population. Before the twentieth century, we worried more about people starving to death than about many other concerns; thus, the American industrial base turned toward food production. We overcame drought and technology was developed to ensure that hunger would be a thing of the past.

Over the past seventy-five years, Americans have produced more and more, bigger and bigger, and better and better food. Naturally, food prices came down, too, so that virtually all Americans have access to a nourishing diet, even if they don't take advantage of this. Differences between what the various economic classes can eat have narrowed. Basically, we can all eat the same things.

We are now faced with a convergence of two problems that has had an enormous impact on our society. One is overfeeding and the other is underactivity. The result is that, as a nation, we have serious public health problems linked to excess weight.

The fast-food industry's success is based on speed plus familiarity. No matter what city you are in, if you go into McDonald's, the Big Mac is going to be the same. You know that you can go into almost any food store and find "good food." Whether it is good for you or not is another question. It certainly is edible and untainted. You don't have to worry because the food industry is so regulated that any violations are page-one news.

The primary concern of Americans is no longer food but occupational success and money matters. The two-paycheck family must spend less time on food preparation. Often the priority is speed, not value, when it comes to food.

Food preparation today is especially simple. You open the freezer, throw the food on the stove or in the microwave, and it is ready to eat. Your primary personal concern is no longer whether what you eat is going to kill you on the basis of toxicity but that you have to deal with your boss tomorrow, or you have to get a report done, or you have to get it to Cincinnati today.

The overall emphasis of society is on speed and on getting things done. Federal Express started with overnight delivery but that became too slow, so now it's Zap Mail. So, as much as we understand diet's role in our overall public health, it's an issue that is difficult to attack for several reasons.

BEATING THE DIET/STRESS–FAST TRACK CONNECTION: SLOW BUT PERMANENT CHANGES

How do we get people to integrate the new attitudes about diet into modern life-styles? For example, how do you tell people in stress situations to fit their diet into an overall preventive and risk-reducing medical program?

The answer, as far as diet in modern America goes, is that good food is simple. As you will learn in Chapter Six, a balanced diet does not have to be a mystery. You don't have to become an expert in nutrition to eat a balanced diet—you must simply master a few easy-to-learn facts and concepts. You do have to make a commitment to a balanced diet, however.

Our notion of a "balanced" diet is so overinflated with calories, vitamins, and minerals that even if many people reduced their calorie intake by 33 percent, malnutrition would likely still never appear.

The diet answers are most often individual ones geared to specific needs, which is unfortunate, because we are all looking for quick cures. And diet change is the toughest kind. The risks from being overweight can't even be demonstrated by using a device like the blood pressure cuff. Few people believe the scale, which is often not immediately relevant to the risks involved. The individual nature of risk reduction is also one reason why we are writing an "interactive" book like *Beat the Odds*.

One example, however, of dealing with the problem of diet as it relates to today's life-style-induced risk factors can be found in the story of a Healthstyle program we ran.

One of our most successful groups was at a factory in Lowell, Massachusetts. We have treated fifteen employees there, and they have all made major changes in their diet and smoking behavior. We returned every three months for a few years to reinforce the changes they had made. I personally went up there every six months or so to give the group a little pep talk and to answer any questions about specific health concerns.

We always try to teach people that they are not going into a temporary program or embarking on a three-week diet. Rather, they will gradually be developing permanent changes in their eating habits through methods described more fully in Chapter Six.

Recently, when we went back to Lowell, the first questions we were asked by these very successful men were, "When can I stop doing this? When can I go back to living the way I did before?" These questions continued, despite all we had said about permanent changes. "When are you going to have a magic pill that is like Drano and washes out my arteries so I don't have to worry about this anymore?" This response to dietary changes is directly related to the presence of both so much good nutrition and so much stress that we always want a quick cure.

What we say to people then is also the main message of *Beat the Odds* and all risk-reduction programs.

We are looking for you to make permanent changes in your behavior. But we don't expect you to become a recluse. We want you to go out on Sunday afternoon with your family for a drive and have an ice cream sundae, but to do it only once a week or, better yet, once a month. We will have achieved a major triumph if, before we met, you ate a pint of ice cream in front of the TV every night. You've overcome the basic problem if you are now having a piece of fruit or a bowl of popcorn in front of the TV.

EXECUTIVE STRESS CAN INCREASE THE ODDS

What roles do personal and professional stress and our modern society's high-tech living standards play in our dietary problems? We see trends for the better in the executive suite and in the advertising for health clubs and exotic foods, but these are still only trends.

The stress/society risk factor and its relationship to diet is especially important to understand now, since virtually everybody in this country knows that the food they are going to get is "good" (i.e., nontoxic).

Certainly anyone who reads about the potential risks engendered by diet and stress (along with all the others mentioned here) should pay attention to his or her own condition, right? But we also know, because of the asymptomatic nature of risk, that most people don't. We know that as doctors we should provide better teaching and we know we should provide the best possible information so that our patients can choose successful strategies to reduce risk.

But still, often we don't succeed, even with those *most* at risk. How do we reach these stressed-out, fast track–type people who understand the issues, read the workbooks, are motivated, but still don't make changes?

Why do some who are in the fast track and in the same boat as their colleagues nonetheless fail in their attempts to reduce health risks? One example of this is a former patient of mine who was once the vice president for finance of a major corporation, but got laid off when the industry underwent a shakeout.

Despite the fact that he soon landed another job, he was humiliated by the fact that he was now underemployed. During the year, despite few problems at the new job, he began to smoke and drink excessively. He became depressed. Quitting these habits was clearly not high on his list of priorities, despite all the efforts we made to convince him through professional counseling that his life could get better.

Soon after landing that new job, he died of overwhelming pneumonia. He could never perceive himself as being in control of his life. He could see nothing positive in his immediate environment, and it contributed to his poor health behavior. The fact is, a person must *value* life and good health in order to go to the trouble and effort to obtain it.

Look, though, at how *successful* people respond to the same type of issue.

In the last year, I've seen in my office two senior vice-presidents and two corporate presidents of major high-tech companies. They have all been long-term executives in the industry; all have held prestige jobs at a variety of other companies. I was struck by the fact that these men, who have been on the fastest track in America's most rapidly growing industry, are very knowledgeable about nourishment. They know what they eat, they exercise every day, they are very conscious of their weight, and none of them smoke.

These people are the ones who became patients before they became sick. They understand that their success at work makes their health valuable to them. They have learned to do what is necessary in order to succeed at their life's missions.

I recently saw a 35-year-old executive on a similar fast track—except this executive had hypertension. The message I had to deliver to him was simple: "Hey, do you like what you're doing? Are you happy? Are you where you thought you'd be fifteen years ago?"

He answered, as do many executives, "I like my job. Sure it's stressful and hard work, but I thrive on it."

The only answer to a response like that is, "Then why do you want to throw it away? Why do you want to die early by virtue of your life-style?"

"What happens if you have a heart attack and survive the heart attack?" I often ask these businesspeople. "The answer is that you are immediately off the fast track. If you are one of five corporate VPs in line to be president and you have your heart attack at age forty-two, you are off the presidential track. So why not introduce the life-style changes I am suggesting to you now at a time when you can continue to be on the fast track."

You'd be surprised at how this sort of "health blackmail" works on certain types of executives—stress-ridden, but health-educated overachievers. These fast-moving executives are a part of society that we must treat differently in order to get them to reduce risks. Their failure to reduce risks will result in great economic loss to them. Their "buttons" are different, and a rational appeal often doesn't work.

For a lot of our fathers, the tradition was that work was drudgery that you had to go through to provide food and security for your family. Work, our fathers told us, is what you do so that when you get through with it, you can have a few beers and go out with your buddies. Or go home and watch TV and live happily ever after.

But to today's executives, work has become much like a lover. They work not only to produce for their families but also because they love the idea of succeeding.

Once they succeed, however, they become trapped. They get the big cars they want, but it only becomes a nuisance to have these cars serviced and fixed.

I have lots of patients who, when they come back from a vacation, stop by the office on the way home from the airport, to get their mail. Even the night before they go back to work they're working.

There *must* be some balance to your life, no matter how consuming your job is. If you say to me, "I am not able to take off at lunchtime and go play squash, my day is too busy," I'll say, "Fine, do it at seven in the morning. Ride a stationary bicycle while you are reading financial reports. You have to allow yourself to put health on the list, and when you decide where to put it, it can't be anywhere but at the top of that list."

Once you've made your health a priority, there is one more step to take. Now that you have considered the current state of health risk reduction in our society, the various roles we play, and the various effects of the economy and modern life, your next undertaking is to follow the strategies we set up in this book to meet the challenges in your own *Beat the Odds Health Profile*.

Strategies to Beat the Odds

Someone once said: "All life is basically 8:5 against." So, if you want to beat the odds, you have to practice health from the earliest possible age; you have to develop lifelong positive health habits. If, however, you find you're now at risk, don't—we repeat, *don't*—just give up and have another candy bar. Most of our health-related problems are correctable—some partially, some totally. And remember, the sooner you start practicing health, the sooner you'll be on your way back.

Few of think about being healthy until we're actually sick. Healthy people rarely remember just how bad they felt the last time they were sick. In fact, we confuse not being sick with being healthy. This is a dangerous attitude for it leads to lazy health habits. And laziness can lead to disaster.

By now, you have some idea of the nature of your own personal health risks. You may be a candidate for a heart attack, or a stroke. You may be a Type A person (see Chapter Eight), ready to explode from anger stress. You may be inadvertently inviting cancer. What follows in this book are strategies—personal strategies that will aid you in reducing your health risks and help you beat the odds and live longer.

Everyone must set goals to obtain good health. The most important thing is to make certain simple, common-sense life-style changes, such as improving your diet, exercising regularly, quitting smoking, controlling your weight, and coping with stress.

Of course, you won't be able to make all of these changes at once. You don't have to move to a monastery, have your jaw wired shut, or radically alter your environment. Nobody fails more quickly than a "born-again" dieter using a quick-fix strategy. People fail at most goal-oriented strategies for one major reason—they reach their goals too easily. That's right—once they've lost those 20 or 30 pounds, or have gone to the health club for a few months to exercise, they lose motivation. They fail because all they think of is their single-minded diet goal or their very specific exercise program, rather than actually altering and making permanent changes in their health habits.

Goals should be set up that help you make permanent changes in your life-style, not simply to lose 15 pounds or run 26 miles. The result of focusing on losing 15 pounds or running a marathon is that once you've done it, you've *finished*. There's nowhere else to go.

Set goals that enhance your life-style. For example, each week— rain, sunshine, snow, or sleet—block out two to four hours and devote that time to fitness. Or decide to eliminate 500 calories a day from your diet. But the key is to think in terms of permanence. *Every* week you will exercise two to four hours a week. *Every* day you'll eliminate those calories. Every day, every week, every year for the rest of your life.

These long-term strategies will *change the way you approach your health*. They are the beginning of a whole new way of life.

THE FIRST TEN WAYS

Here are several general but immediate ways to improve your overall health. Consider them as basic building blocks before you go on to the specific strategies for your own risk factors that follow this chapter.

1. *Join or Form a Good Health Network:* In some ways, this may be your most important strategy. Announce to the world, or at the very least to your family and friends, that you are going to beat the odds. You're going to be following certain plans or steps in the next few months that will alter your life and may affect theirs. Find a "buddy" —your wife, a friend, or colleague—to talk with about your plan

and, if possible, to help or join you. If you're part of a good health network, you'll always have other people to turn to if you feel that you're slipping and need a confidence booster.

As part of this health network, hook up with a good doctor who can teach you about exercise or nutrition. Find a doctor who can recommend a solid program to help you stop smoking or any other expert assistance you need. See Chapter Five for specific ways to evaluate and choose a physician.

2. *Learn the Facts:* No one beats the odds with his head in the sand. Any new skill, whether it's improving health habits or driving a car, requires learning the "how to's" of the activity. If, for example, you want to lose weight, learning about the caloric content of foods is more important than following a diet sheet. You'll be able to make selections from a wider array of foods once you know about food values.

Learning the facts does not, by the way, mean that you have to become an expert—just an informed participant. If you are at risk for heart disease, you should know that more than 600,000 of your fellow Americans die from this disease annually. Or that the more coronary risk factors you have, the greater your chances of a heart attack—the increase is proportional. Solid, correct information is the best motivator for good health behavior.

3. *Admit That You Are at Risk:* Diseases such as strokes or heart attacks just don't happen to other people. Think about friends or relatives you know who actually suffer from what you are at risk of suffering. How has it affected their lives? Are they still independent? Are they dead? Has it hurt their family lives? Think about the effects of ignoring the risks. Then think about the benefits of reducing the risks. The choice isn't too hard. Certainly, ignoring a coronary risk, for example, won't make it vanish even if you have no symptoms at the moment. (Some 55 percent of all heart attack victims die before reaching a hospital. The first symptom of this often preventable illness is death!) *Admit you could get seriously ill, even die, because you're at heightened risk—then decide you're going to do something about reducing that risk.*

4. *Make a Commitment and Stick to It:* This is another crucial step if you are going to change your health habits. To begin with, choose a

reachable goal that you can achieve in a reasonable time. Pin a sign up over your desk that says I'M CHANGING THE WAY I EAT. I'M GOING TO CHANGE THE WAY I EAT AND I WILL LOSE WEIGHT IN FOUR WEEKS. Write down exactly how you're going to get to that goal. Tell someone— tell everyone—especially your kids. They'll be more than happy to tell you when you're slipping! Write down when you succeed and write down when you screw up. Feel guilty when you slip (you *should* feel guilty), but recognize that you are entitled to rewards for good behavior. We're not in trouble when we eat an *occasional* ice cream cone. We're in trouble when we sit down in front of the TV and eat ice cream every night!

No matter what happens, don't give up—tinker with the approach and change it until it works. Make improved health a lifelong goal.

5. *Exercise Regularly:* Exercise should be a part of everyone's life. It's not just recreation but a necessary health behavior for everyone! The types of exercises you do should be discussed with your doctor, but as a guide, keep in mind that it should be something you can adopt as a lifelong recreation. It helps if it's fun and challenging as well as healthy. It can be walking, jogging, swimming, biking, tennis, racquetball, or whatever, as long as it's enjoyable rather than a chore. The old "it's gotta hurt to make a difference" theory has turned many people off exercise. What is important is to make sure that you exercise vigorously, working up a sweat for thirty minutes at least three or four times a week.

To be effective, the concept of exercise as a health measure should be exactly the same as personal hygiene. Certainly, you don't feel right if you don't brush your teeth each day. That's how you should feel about exercise. Once exercise is a habit, you don't decide whether to do it, you just do it.

Of course, you should also consider other ways of beating your odds through exercise. Approach your body as a machine that needs to keep moving. For example, when you drive to work or the market, park your car at the far end of the lot and walk; use stairs instead of an elevator. How many times have you cruised the parking lot at the mall looking for a space close to the store? Isn't it an ironic waste of time and health?

The value of exercise should not be news to any American in 1985. We're flooded daily with data about the benefits of fitness. In fact, a recent study conducted at the Harvard Medical School clearly proved that even mild exercise reduces the risk of heart attack. Yet all too few of us connect fitness with health. Being fit is not a cosmetic exercise. Your fitness level isn't related only to your dress or jacket size, or how nice you look—it's directly connected to how long you'll live. Being fit is not a guarantee of good health, but it is an integral part of health.

6. *Eat a Sensible Diet to Control Weight:* Good nutrition is another one of the obvious strategies that many of us ignore. For certain people with a high risk of heart disease, this may mean eliminating fat, cholesterol, and saturated oils from the diet, or avoiding whole milk dairy products, red meat, sugar, alcohol, etcetera. For others, good nutritional habits may mean turning away from candy to veggies—not always an easy task.

The human body is a remarkable machine, able to run on a wide range of fuels. As we have evolved, food has been scarce most of the time, so our bodies developed the ability to run for long times between fill-ups. Now, ironically, many of our illnesses are related to an overabundance of fuel, along with labor-saving convenience devices, which cut down on exercise.

It is true that most people can still eat pretty much what they want and suffer few ill effects. But if your genetic predisposition causes your cholesterol or triglyceride levels to rise when you eat too much of certain foods, then you have to learn to control your eating behavior and, more important, be willing to take these steps immediately.

Most Americans simply need to eat less. It is likely you don't need all the calories you consume. But to cut down, you have to find a new eating style that you can be comfortable with for a long time—forever. This book contains many strategies for weight loss and diet change that work. Use them. Try them. You'll get by with them.

7. *Have a Physical Exam:* You should see your doctor for a physical exam. The doctor should check your blood pressure and take blood samples to check your levels of HDL, cholesterol, triglycerides, blood sugar, and other chemistries to mark your progress. The only way to determine certain problems that put you at risk—and high blood pressure is a particularly dangerous one—is to see a doctor for a thorough exam. You can also watch for Health Fair Screening Programs at your local mall and stop in—this is a good way to get a quick check on your blood pressure. You'll find more detailed infor-

mation on blood-pressure control in Chapter Seven. But the place to measure certain kinds of success when you begin to practice health is in the doctor's office, where your physician can give you a thorough checkup, get to know your problems, and monitor the changes you have made.

8. *Quit Smoking:* People know that smoking is bad for the heart and lungs. *The only acceptable level of smoking is zero.* Because if you aren't at risk now, smoking will lead you to risk heart disease or cancer—it's guaranteed. No matter what anyone tells you, smoking is a terrible habit. It's probably the most important public health menace in the country. We've outlined many strategies in Chapter Nine that will enable you to join the smokeless generation. Think of your improved health, not to mention all the money you'll be saving. Remember, even one cigarette is bad—so quit for good! Today!

9. *Learn to Cope:* Not all stress is bad. We sometimes need stress to get motivated to do things. But figure out where stress is affecting you adversely. Either solve your problems by learning to relax or else put yourself right in line for serious illness. If stress controls your life, you must take charge of it. Don't let it rule you. In Chapter Eight, you'll find many many specific suggestions on ways to cope with stress, but the most important is your overall attitude. Be positive. Work through your problems—either get beyond them or learn to live with them. Often your attitudes toward your goals affect how well you cope. You can control stress by changing your attitudes about life, setting realistic goals, and practicing the techniques described in Chapter Eight. Another general rule for stress control is let it all hang out. Don't keep your feelings and problems bottled up—share your problems with others in your household. Stress doesn't go away, but it shouldn't be the boss. Take charge of your environment as part of your good health program. Responding to stress with anger is particularly harmful.

10. *Check Yourself:* Don't fool yourself—make sure your health program is working. Sometimes, simply working toward a goal isn't enough. You have to make sure you're working in the right way. If you have to control high blood pressure, for example, consider a home monitoring device. Have blood tests done every six months to see if you've lowered your cholesterol or triglyceride levels. If you're

not making progress, it's okay to change your health program. The important thing is to find what works for you.

A Final Note: There are no guaranteed ways to good health. Adopting good health habits is an individual task. Use your *Beat the Odds Health Profile* as an indicator to form a basic health plan that works for you. Once you begin, you will probably see some immediate results. Perhaps you'll lose weight, or feel better. You certainly will feel better about being in control of your own life.

But only time will really tell whether you've begun to practice health. You will want to have regular progress checks. Then you will really see if you've begun to beat the odds.

Let's Get Started!

INCLUDE A DOCTOR IN YOUR RISK-REDUCTION NETWORK

A key aspect of learning to reduce risk is the proper selection of a doctor. After all, you choose a money manager very carefully, based on his or her performance for others. You choose a lawyer based on qualification and competence. If you are going to be able to learn about risk reduction and succeed in that effort, you should consider the choice of doctor as a crucial, life-saving step.

You need to have a good doctor as one of your network of important people. Just as your lawyer, accountant, pharmacist, and minister know you, you should also have a doctor who knows who you are, who knows you as a person with health risk factors.

But how do we justify this in view of the fact that we have also said that doctors don't do a good job of educating people? And that doctors don't have the time to educate people?

What we are really suggesting here is that you choose your doctor to play a special role in your life. First of all, you need the doctor as an evaluator of symptoms. You should be able to call up your doctor and say, "I have had pain in my shoulder for the last two weeks." The doctor pulls out your record and says, "Five years ago you complained about pain in your shoulder for two weeks. We just put you on some aspirin and it went away." This is one kind of role that your doctor should play. But it is not necessarily the only role.

Is the doctor's role to be a kind of supertechnician? Is that what the physician has evolved into?

No, because despite the recognition that people can develop their own risk-reduction strategies, many people make changes in their lives only because they feel that their doctor cares that they make the changes. The key words here are the proprietary "their doctor."

All too often a patient will come into my office, and I will say, "I notice you haven't lost any weight." And the patient will apologize and say, "Gee, Doc, I'm *sorry* but I haven't been able to."

What that tells me is that a lot of the motivation for making behavioral change occurs when there is somebody watching you, somebody monitoring your changes. Somebody who will *care* that you have changed.

Although we would like to believe that people make life-style changes simply because of the rational view that they are going to live longer if they do so, that just is not so.

To some extent, your doctor could serve as a mentor or even a judge. When I tell patients how delighted I am that they have reduced their cholesterol levels, I *am* delighted. My view is that I may have had an input into that change. I am delighted that they are able to gain control of this issue and make the changes—and that serves as a very strong reinforcer to the patients.

HOW TO JUDGE "THE JUDGE"

If you go to a doctor and he or she tells you your blood pressure is up a bit but you don't need to do anything about it, the doctor may be saying that because of a strong belief that you don't need to do anything about it. But the doctor may also be saying, "I've got fifty other people sitting in the waiting room, and for me to stop and explain to this patient about blood pressure medicine is going to waste my time. The patient is not going to get sick this month from that high blood pressure, so I will just get this person out of my office."

There certainly are good doctors around. But unfortunately there are also lousy doctors, who succeed in life only because they know when to refer their patients to somebody else. Their stock in trade is establishing a supposedly great warm relationship with their patients. When their patients get sick, these doctors may not know exactly what is wrong, but they have established an army of consultants who can take care of the problems.

Then how do you distinguish between a good doctor who will treat you properly himself and one who can only send you along to someone else?

HOW TO SELECT A PHYSICIAN

First you have to define what you want the physician for.

Let's assume you want a physician to provide adult medical care for you and/or your spouse. The physician you choose should be prepared to spend forty-five to sixty minutes with you during an initial evaluation. This evaluation should include questions of personal historical significance. (Some physicians ask you to fill out forms ahead of time.)

These questions should include: types of illnesses you had as a child; types of operations, allergies, diseases your parents and other close family members have suffered; and your occupational status. You should also be asked about diet, alcohol, exercise, tobacco use. The doctor should want to know something about your psychological makeup even before he does a relatively thorough physical exam. My own personal view is that it is much more important to do a thorough historical examination initially, than a thorough physical exam. This is vital for identification of your health risks.

There are a number of things included in a "complete physical," including an eye examination, exam for glaucoma, prostate exams, examinations of the distal colon through sigmoidoscopy.

If you are a woman, your physician should be competent to do more than just a gynecological exam. If your doctor doesn't take into consideration cholesterol levels, smoking behavior, blood pressure, etcetera, but only deals with gynecology, make sure that you are referred to a family practitioner or internist.

For most people, the general practitioner geared toward preventive issues is probably the person that you want to deal with. The primary-care internist who is also devoted to prevent issues is also someone you want to deal with.

Where a doctor went to school, or how the doctor performed on certain examinations is not important to me. Rather, I think that what actually goes on in the office—how much time is spent with the patient, how organized the office is on prevention issues—is more important than whether someone is a general practitioner or certified sub-subspecialist. And I also think that word of mouth—what the experiences of your friends has been—is a factor to consider.

The doctor who fits this bill doesn't have to be in a large medical center in a major urban center, either.

I was once on a panel with a family doctor, Bill Manahan, who lives in a small town—Mankato, Minnesota—and I would let him take care of me any day of the week. He had learned how to do manipulations from a chiropractor to help relieve the suffering of his patients. He had a social worker and a nutritionist working along with him in his office to take care of the things that I think physicians are incapable of doing alone. He was very interested in people's diets and other life-style elements, and how they affected their risk of disease.

He is wonderful. He struck me as one of the best doctors I've ever encountered. Whether I had lupus, diffuse pulmonary interstitial fibrosis, or severe cardiac disease, I would trust this man to make sure I got into the right hands. And I would feel very happy with him helping me on life-style issues.

HOW TO KNOW THE PHYSICIAN YOU WANT

What kind of doctor do you want? Do you want someone who will sit and explain each illness in great detail? Or do you want someone who will just reassure you and tell you that "you are going to be all right if you do what I say"?

Some people require doctors who are personable and nice and sweet, and others are very happy with authoritarian, parental figures.

You need to answer your questions before you look at their qualifications.

There are some professional questions that are important in the choice of a doctor. For example, the hospitals where the doctor works is of major importance. If the hospital has a poor reputation, it may well be that this doctor is not viewed very highly by his or her colleagues and can't get on the staff of a good hospital. That needs to be taken into consideration.

You will want to know who the physician would refer you to for the more common ailments which you are more likely to develop in your life. Since two-thirds of us are going to die of heart disease and stroke, who is the neurologist or cardiologist that the doctor uses for referral? To which medical centers does he refer people for cancer therapy? Those kinds of questions should be answered.

Be familiar with your doctor's fees and what the general fee schedules in your area are. Make sure that your doctor will discuss this issue with you. Learn about insurance coverage. Don't let money issues spoil an otherwise good relationship.

We are no longer in an era when one doctor can take care of everything. Rather, you need one doctor, the primary physician, who can serve as the clearinghouse and the triage. Once you have that person in place and you are comfortable with the hospital affiliation plus such matters as personal characteristics—amount of time spent with patients, fees, attitudes toward house calls and telephone calls—then you can depend on this doctor when other kinds of expertise are needed.

WHEN TO SEE THE DOCTOR

Are you an adult male who has never had any particularly serious ailments and whose family history is benign? This means:

- parents still living
- grandparents lived to be over 65
- no unusual illnesses running in the family
- never had any particular serious health problems

Some 80 percent of American males at age 35 should have a careful physical examination and identify an internist or primary-care GP to establish a relationship with, as we've described.

Before age 35, the typical American male may not have developed blood pressure elevation, and his cholesterol levels may still be low. These things tend to rise to their adult levels by age 35.

Women in the same age category who have seen a gynecologist regularly and had annual Pap smears might also consider going to an internist or family doctor for a complete evaluation. Often what has happened is that your family doctor may have delivered your baby but may *not* have stopped to measure your cholesterol levels, to talk to you about controlling your blood pressure, or to discuss the effects of smoking. It's at this point in your life that you need to get your doctors lined up.

How often should someone see a physician? Of course, recommendations vary, and they increase with age. It is my own view that in the decade between ages 30 and 40, all people should have a complete physical exam. An EKG should be recorded in their charts somewhere to serve as a baseline. People should also have a chest X ray recorded in their chart, again as a baseline.

If you are a smoker, chest X rays should be done every few years. If you are a nonsmoker, every decade. People in their forties should be examined rectally with a sigmoidoscope and have urinalysis and blood tests performed. If you have normal cholesterol levels, or low cholesterol and low triglyceride levels, then every five years should be often enough to have these things measured.

If, at age 35, you don't have any hypertension, elevated cholesterol levels, or diabetes, and you have a family history of longevity, then your risk of dying prematurely of heart disease is very, very low. Yet a good doctor can still help you factor in other possibilities, such as occupational exposure or environmental threats that you may not be aware of.

It is still the case that most of us are going to die of heart attack and stroke even without taking risks like smoking or poor dietary behavior. What we are talking about is shifting that death to age 80 from age 50, by not having a variety of risk factors.

GETTING THE MOST OUT OF YOUR DOCTOR

Before seeing your doctor—even if it's a first visit—take the time to write down exactly what has been bothering you, if anything. Don't feel that you must exaggerate your symptoms to justify your visit, but don't underestimate them either. Be specific when describing your problem; for example, is the pain sharp and needlelike, or is it dull and throbbing? When you lie down does the pain go away? Is there more pain after physical activity?

Also write down any medications you may be taking, the dosage strength and how often you take the medication, and the reason for taking the drug. Remember to record even over-the-counter medications, such as the kind you may take for colds, allergies, or pain. Vitamins count, too.

Write down any conditions, such as high blood pressure or ulcers, that you may have now or have had in the past. Note any family history of diabetes, heart disease, cancer, or strokes. In addition, it is very important to write down any questions or fears you may have *before* visiting your doctor.

By writing down all this information, you'll help your doctor determine what the problem is, and you'll feel more secure in your doctor's judgment.

When you do visit your doctor, the most important thing is to speak up and ask questions. Your doctor won't know if you don't understand something unless you speak up and tell him or her that you are confused. Don't be embarrassed. After all, this is *your* health and *your* body that the doctor is talking about. If, after you try to communicate better, your doctor still refuses to answer questions, or obviously has a difficult time talking with you, get another doctor whom you *can* talk to.

Insist that a thorough personal and family history be taken during your first visit. If your doctor claims that he or she doesn't have the time to take such a history, say that you don't have the time for this examination. Then get another doctor who will take a proper history.

After visiting your doctor, ask yourself these questions:

- Does your doctor explain what's happening?
- Do you feel comfortable asking questions?
- Does your doctor give you straight answers?
- Will your doctor listen to complaints?
- Does your doctor spend enough time with you?

If you don't like the answers to these questions, then maybe it is time to get another doctor, or at the very least, make your dissatisfaction known.

WHAT ABOUT A SECOND OPINION?

If your doctor tells you that you need surgery, in most instances you shouldn't hesitate to get a second opinion.

First, after your diagnosis, check with your insurance company to see what kind of coverage you have. Some policies will pay for surgery *only* if two opinions confirm the need. Some will even pay for a third "tie-breaker" if the two opinions conflict.

Most surgeons today welcome a second opinion. It helps protect them from malpractice suits later and makes the patient more confident about the surgery. Any surgeon who objects to a second opinion should explain these objections to your satisfaction.

Don't ask your doctor to recommend someone for a second opinion. Choose a second surgeon with no connection to the first. And if you don't know whom to choose, call the national referral service of Cornell University–New York Hospital Hotline (800-522-0036 or 800-631-1220 in New York) for a board-certified surgeon in your area.

SIX

Beating the Heart Odds

WHAT IS HEART DISEASE?

The Cardiovascular System

So far, we've been talking about heart disease and coronary risk factors in a very general way. In this chapter we'll take a closer look at heart disease, and what each coronary risk factor can mean in terms of years lost from your life. In order to understand what heart disease is all about, it's first necessary to look at how a healthy heart and circulatory system works.

The body's cardiovascular system includes the heart, arteries, and veins. The heart is an incredible pumping station, handling more than 100 gallons of blood every hour. Arteries are the vessels that carry blood from the heart to all the organs and tissues of the body. Blood carried in the arteries is rich in oxygen, which all cells need for life and growth. Once blood has given its oxygen to the body's cells and has collected the cells' waste products (such as carbon dioxide), it returns to the heart through the veins. The heart then pumps the blood to the lungs, where it is given a fresh supply of oxygen. From the lungs, the blood goes back to the heart, where it is again pumped throughout the body.

Blood Pressure

Blood pressure is the force of the blood as it flows through the arteries. It is taken in two readings. The first is done when the heart contracts, and is called the *systolic pressure.* A systolic pressure of 100 to 140 is normal. The second reading, the *diastolic pressure,* is taken when the heart relaxes. Normal diastolic readings are between 70 and 90. So, when you hear of a blood pressure of, say, 130 over 80, that means a systolic pressure of 130 and a diastolic pressure of 80. A diagnosis of high blood pressure, also called "hypertension," means that your systolic and/or diastolic readings are above the normal limits. (See Chapter Seven for more detailed information on high blood pressure.)

Coronary Arteries: The Heart's Lifelines

The heart, like all organs, needs blood to nourish its cells and carry away heart-cell wastes. The blood that is pumped in the heart doesn't actually give oxygen to the heart's cells; this is done by blood that reaches the heart through separate "coronary arteries," which surround the heart like a crown (the word "coronary," in fact, comes from *corona,* a Latin word meaning "crown"). The coronary arteries are vitally important to the heart—if one becomes blocked or closes off, part of the heart will die. Blockages come about through a gradual buildup of fatty materials and cholesterol in the arteries. This buildup is called atherosclerosis (also arteriosclerosis).

Atherosclerosis: Clogging of the Arteries

Atherosclerosis takes place over a span of many years. During that time, fat and cholesterol are deposited in the inner walls of arteries. As the deposits build up, the arteries become narrower.

Since the process of building up fatty deposits is slow and gradual, the symptoms of atherosclerosis may take years to show up. And when they do, a person who appeared perfectly healthy may suddenly be stricken with a serious, even fatal condition. Let's look at some of the problems that result from atherosclerosis.

Angina Pectoris (Chest Pains)

Angina results from a reduced flow of blood to the heart. The symptoms are a heaviness, tightness, or squeezing pain in the chest. It is

About Angina Pectoris

1. This kind of chest pain is caused by inadequate blood flow to the heart.
2. It is especially noticeable during exercise, when the heart needs more oxygen but can't get it.
3. The symptoms of angina (heaviness, tightness, or squeezing pain in the chest) can be controlled with drugs. Bypass surgery can also eliminate the symptoms.

especially common during exercise, when the heart muscle needs more oxygen but can't get it because the coronary arteries are partially blocked. These symptoms usually go away if the person rests.

The symptoms of angina can be controlled with various drugs that widen the obstructed arteries, thus decreasing the work of the heart. The surgical technique called coronary artery bypass has also been used to bring relief to people suffering from angina. The technique involves removing a piece of vein from the leg and using it to make connections around the obstructed part of the coronary arteries. These "detours" allow blood to flow freely around the obstructions and deliver their supplies of oxygen to the heart muscle. Bypass surgery is effective in increasing the heart's blood supply; however, if the health habits that contributed to artery damage in the first place aren't dealt with, the angina problems will just come back in time. In other words, even after bypass surgery, a person still has to make changes in his or her health habits.

Heart Attack (a.k.a. Myocardial Infarction, Coronary Thrombosis, or "Coronary")

A heart attack occurs when a portion of the heart muscle suddenly dies from lack of blood and oxygen. This happens when a coronary artery becomes completely closed off. An artery can become blocked either by a large buildup of fatty deposits on the inner walls, or by a blood clot forming on the deposits and plugging the opening. In either case, the lack of blood can cause serious damage to the part of the heart muscle that is fed by the obstructed artery.

A heart attack is most often characterized by chest pain, which may spread to the left arm, shoulders, jaw, or back. Other symptoms include sweating, shortness of breath, nausea, vomiting, and loss of consciousness. The symptoms might disappear and then return min-

About Heart Attacks

1. They are caused by blockage in a coronary artery, so that part of the heart becomes starved for oxygen and dies.
2. The symptoms include extreme chest pain, which spreads to the left arm, shoulders, back, and jaw. Also sweating, shortness of breath, nausea, vomiting, and loss of consciousness may occur.
3. Most heart attack deaths happen before the person gets to the hospital. Don't wait if you have the symptoms of a heart attack—get help immediately.

utes to hours later. More than half of heart attack deaths occur *before* the victim reaches the hospital. In fact, the average victim waits *three hours* before looking for help—and those are three hours that he or she just might not be able to afford. Anyone experiencing the symptoms of a heart attack should *immediately* get medical help—every minute counts.

Sudden Cardiac Death

Sudden cardiac death occurs when the heart of someone with coronary artery disease begins beating ineffectively. Very rapid or irregular heartbeats greatly weaken the pumping action of the heart, so that vital tissues throughout the body become starved for oxygen. Death usually occurs within a few moments of the attack. Sudden cardiac death often strikes people with no other signs of coronary heart disease, and who seem to be in good health.

Stroke

When arteries supplying blood to the brain become blocked or burst from very high pressure, a stroke occurs. A stroke, like a heart attack, can result from fatty deposits closing off an artery, or a blood clot forming on the deposits and sealing the vessel. Some strokes happen because a blood vessel in the brain ruptures. This can occur when a vessel is weakened by atherosclerosis or high blood pressure. A stroke can cause temporary or permanent paralysis, slurred speech, loss of memory, or loss of consciousness. Recovery may be very quick—in a matter of days—or very slow, taking months. Sometimes the dam-

---

About Stroke

1. A stroke is caused by a blockage in an artery that supplies blood to the brain.
2. Symptoms include paralysis, slurred speech, loss of memory, or loss of consciousness, depending on which area of the brain has lost its blood supply.
3. The symptoms may be temporary or permanent.

---

age is irreversible. A major stroke, like a major heart attack, can be a fatal event.

How Widespread Is Atherosclerosis?

Atherosclerosis is one of our nation's major health problems—it leads to more deaths and disabilities than any other disease. Coronary heart disease is especially widespread in this country: Some 640,000 people die each year from it. Of those deaths, 400,000 are sudden or happen unexpectedly. Other complications of atherosclerosis account for about 200,000 deaths a year, 180,000 of these being stroke victims.

The costs of atherosclerotic diseases are staggering: The American Heart Association estimated that in 1981, heart and blood vessel diseases cost the nation *$46 billion* in terms of medical care and productivity losses from disability or death. Most of those costs were the result of coronary heart disease.

The amount of time lost from work and recreation is also enormous. In 1978, atherosclerosis accounted for: 33 million hospital days, 86 million bed days, 21 million work-loss days, and 241 million restricted-activity days. Again, coronary heart disease was in the lead, resulting in: 20 million hospital days, 61 million bed days, 18 million work-loss days, and 184 million restricted-activity days.

LOSING WEIGHT TO REDUCE THE RISK OF HEART DISEASE

According to your particular *Beat the Odds Health Profile,* losing weight may be one way you can prevent or reduce the risk of heart disease. Perhaps over your lifetime or over a number of years, you have developed several health behavior patterns—including poor diet —that have raised the odds against you and for a heart attack. One result is that you are overweight, a serious risk factor that can lead to heart disease and related problems.

This *weight risk* can be reduced. It is possible. But if you eat too much of the wrong foods and exercise too little, the odds will never diminish. You may also have a genetic "program" that compels you to weigh too much, and you'll have to swim against that tide also. If you are at risk because of weight, your eating behavior—either conscious or unconscious—is largely negative. To beat the odds, you're going to have to start thinking positively and exchange your current eating habits for new, healthier habits.

Despite the fact that countless diets appear each year, losing weight is not easy. There are hundreds of methods that mix folklore and science. There are as many claims and counterclaims about certain methods of weight loss as there are experts. But the simple fact is this, losing weight permanently is never, ever an easy task. It will require enormous personal energy and a lifetime commitment. *But this ability is not beyond your capability if you are diligent and apply yourself.*

First, I simply ask you to believe that losing weight to reduce heart risk has nothing to do with "going on a diet." In fact, I ask you to accept that weight loss and dieting, as we know it, generally have very little to do with each other. I ask you to realize that changing your dietary habits will include a very difficult task—learning to not eat instinctively. From now on, every time you eat, you'll have to first ask yourself, Do I really want to do this? But as you learn, you will replace a bad habit—unhealthy eating behavior—with new, better habits. And then you will be on your way to good health.

LEARNING ABOUT FOOD VALUES

Losing weight to help your heart means you must learn a little about nutrition. You will not have to become an expert. You will, however, have to make an effort to understand the simple principles that govern nourishment. This isn't too difficult.

For example, you should know that *all* food contains only three kinds of energy sources: carbohydrates, proteins, and fats. As you learn how to judge the calories in your foods, you'll see how easy it is to decide which foods you want to eat and when.

Therefore, there is only one diet for losing weight. It may consist of

What's the Connection Between Diet and Heart Disease?

As far as your heart is concerned, you really are what you eat—the amount of food and the kinds of food you eat greatly affect the health of your heart and blood vessels (in medical terms, your *cardiovascular system*). When you eat more than you need, you gain weight. And when you're overweight, your blood pressure tends to be higher than it should be.

If you're overeating, you're also probably eating too much fat—which causes your body to make too much cholesterol, a waxy substance that narrows your blood vessels. Once your blood vessels get plugged, your heart, brain, and other organs can become deprived of oxygen. This can lead to heart attack and stroke.

Studies have shown that people who eat a lot of saturated animal fat and oils have higher blood cholesterol levels and suffer more from heart disease than those who eat a diet low in saturated animal fats and oils. So we believe that if a high-fat/high-cholesterol diet can bring a high risk of heart attack, then changing to a low-fat/low-cholesterol diet can bring you down into a lower risk group—which is what this chapter is about.

You'll learn how to change your daily eating habits so that you take in less fats and oils, less cholesterol, and fewer calories.

certain strategies—mixing low calories, low fat, and high fiber to bring certain chemistries into balance—but essentially, there is only one single way to lose weight for reduction of heart risk: Eat fewer calories.

As a person at risk for heart disease, you'll learn why there are several direct links between your health and the values found in our commons foods, such as cholesterol levels, sodium, fiber, or various types of carbohydrates.

In Chapter Twelve you can learn more about these risk factors and nutrition. If you read this section you'll have done more for yourself than a week of fasting.

CAN YOU LOSE WEIGHT FOREVER?

"Going on a diet" is not the way to lose weight permanently. And it's certainly not the way to reduce the risk of heart disease. Yet most overweight people say "I'm dieting," or "I'm going on the [insert latest fad] diet," or "I've got to lose 20 pounds before the wedding next month."

Why is dieting so popular?

Well, one reason is many people can lose weight temporarily and often quite easily. It isn't very difficult to drop 5 or 10 pounds in a few weeks. There are people with "thin" and "fat" wardrobes. These people—all of them—are fooling themselves. They aren't actually controlling their weight. They are temporarily altering their appearance. Such crash or "cosmetic" dieting may be very dangerous.

Quick diets are also popular because they avoid the real issue: losing weight and keeping it off.

This is the most important news in this chapter: The only way to take weight off and keep it off is to make basic life-style changes, replacing current —perhaps negative—habits with new ones. This activity is called behavior modification. We'll come back to this a little later on as we develop several specific strategies for lowering your risk of heart disease through weight loss. But for now, begin reducing your risk with these steps:

STRATEGY

TAKE THE FOOD TEST

Take the food test: Weight is always lost by burning more calories than you take in. How many calories do you consume each day? To find out:

• Start carrying a small spiral notebook with you. Record each and every morsel of food you eat and drink each day for three days: two weekdays and one weekend day. Be honest! No one else is going to read this but you. Be as accurate as possible as you list the sizes of food portions. You may want to buy a food scale to learn about portion size.

• Buy a fifty-cent calorie counter in the supermarket and total how many calories you consume. Don't ignore snacks—little bites here and there just to "tide you over." Don't forget beverages, either soft or alcoholic.

• Buy a good scale—an electronic digital scale. Get used to weighing yourself every day. *Don't hide the scale, keep it in a conspicuous place.* You'll see that your weight fluctuates because of fluids or food taken in. By using the scale you'll have some perspective on where your weight is at all times. You'll think about it. You'll see the consequences of indulgences. You'll also start your days stimulated to eat less. Once you are at the weight range you want to be in for a reasonable period of time, you'll even be able to have overeating periods with less guilt.

THE ACCOUNTING

With your eating accounting in front of you, begin to look for a pattern.

• You'll be able to gauge how many calories per day you eat.

• By checking the charts in this chapter, you can see the "value" of foods that you normally eat; you can judge whether they are high in fats and contribute to heart risk.

• Can you see immediately where you can cut a certain amount of calories each day without too much trouble? Think about this for the future. Some meals have been enjoyable and associated with friends and family; other eating may have been routine, out of vending machines, and easily skipped.

• You should also be able to see *how* you eat each week. Do you nibble? Do you eat twice a day, three times?

The reason for learning about your specific eating patterns is that you will want to change them *as little as possible*. Most so-called diets —especially the fad-of-the-week diets—simply force you, the peg, into a new and different food consumption hole.

If, for example, you never eat breakfast, and some fad diet you are considering says "you must eat breakfast," you're already taking in calories you wouldn't normally have. There's no "magic gain" from eating breakfast. About 25 percent of us aren't hungry at seven a.m., so why eat?

• With this accounting you can *identify* your natural dietary pattern or "style." Then you can fit better choices of foods into that pattern. Keep this information aside for a moment while we consider the next step in reducing risks through weight loss.

STRATEGY

THE EXAM

The next, obvious step is to look in the mirror and decide how much weight you want to lose, right?

No! Absolutely not!

How much weight you need to lose can only be decided in view of the real level of your risk for heart disease. You're reading this chapter because you know that your food choices need changing and you are at some level of risk for a heart attack. Instead, the next step is to determine exactly how much that risk is by examining your blood chemistry. Your weight loss goal may be to bring your cholesterol to normal. This may happen long before your weight falls to a "thin" level.

A PHYSICAL EXAM

• Arrange to have a thorough physical examination that includes a complete profile of your blood chemistry. If you are between 35 and 55 years old, it's vital to tell your doctor that you want certain tests. These include: white blood cell count, hemoglobin, hematocrit, calcium level, phosphorus level, glucose level, BUN (blood/urea/nitrogen), creatinine, uric acid level, cholesterol count, triglyceride count, HDL:cholesterol ratio, total protein level, albumin, globulin, alkaline phosphorus, liver function, and sodium, potassium, chloride, and carbon dioxide levels. *Note:* Cholesterol levels should be between 140 and 225. Anything higher or lower is cause for concern.

• The amount of weight you want to lose will be determined by the results of these tests, especially the blood chemistry levels. You'll have reached the correct weight for you when your blood chemistry is normal. *This is the only measure of weight level that really counts.* The reason why going on a diet fails is that people set lost poundage as a goal, rather than healthy levels of cholesterol, triglycerides, etcetera.

Let's look a little more closely at this idea, especially since it's a lot easier to understand going from size 12 to size 7 than a cholesterol count ratio. How do changing blood values replace the traditional concept of dieting?

Remember, we said that foods can be considered combinations of carbohydrates, fats, and protein. Saturated fats, however, contribute directly to increased cholesterol levels, which you know raise the odds against you.

Remember that fats have twice as many calories per gram as protein and carbohydrates. As a result, any change in food intake that stresses eating fewer fats will bring about a reduction in weight. *And* it will also bring about a simultaneous reduction of cholesterol and triglycerides. You will automatically lose weight by lowering your cholesterol levels—and shift the odds back in your favor.

If you are not overweight but still have high cholesterol levels, you will cut down anyway on certain kinds of foods that have saturated animal fat, substituting, for example, vegetable oil and foods higher in protein and complex carbohydrates. In both cases, risk has been trimmed. Not every overweight person has a heart risk. If you've normalized your blood fat but are still overweight, you've still beat the odds!

LET'S RECAP

So far, you've taken account of how much you eat and seen what kinds of foods you normally eat, gaining some insight into your eating patterns.

And, most important, you've learned that a permanent, realistic method of reducing risk is finding out which blood chemistry risk factors are out of line. *Your weight reduction goal is actually achieved by getting those blood counts into the normal range.*

STRATEGY

WHAT DO WE MEAN BY DIET REWARDS?

Okay, let's go on and improve our eating behavior. Take a minute and start to think a little bit more about what we really mean when we talk about "a diet."

As a noun, the dictionary says that a diet is "food and drink regularly provided or consumed. Habitual nourishment." It is also defined as "the kind and amount of food prescribed for a person . . . for a special reason." As a verb, it means "to cause to eat sparingly or according to prescribed rules."

So everyone is on a diet. If you eat, you have "a diet." Why, then, do Diets, with a capital D, fail? In fact, almost everyone who "goes on a diet" regains their original weight in a year or so. This is because if you are overweight, your so-called normal eating behavior is really overeating for you. Others could eat the same amount and remain thin, but for your biological thermostat—your metabolism—the amount you eat is excessive.

For most people, to go on a diet means they "undereat" for a certain period of time to reach a goal. They maintain that "goal weight" for a while on a diet and then become bored, lose interest and/or motivation, and return to their old diet. After all, once you've reached a goal, what do you do next? Most people go out and overeat as a reward!

So, when you look at your diet account, think in terms of making permanent changes in your food choices at the same time that you reform your eating habits, rather than diet.

With this attitude, you don't have to set a goal of losing 10 or 50 pounds. Your reward will be not having a heart attack. As you learn which foods to eat less of (not avoid for the rest of your life), your chances of success will grow.

THE PRIZE

Many dieters also reward themselves with a "prize" when they lose weight. This is a mistake, because you don't ever complete the task if you've changed your eating behavior. As you lose weight by eating differently, you *will* be rewarded, but in nontraditional, far more important ways. For example, your blood chemistry will begin to show the changes almost immediately. After only a few months of changed eating habits, you'll be able to take blood tests again and see the difference.

It's true that it's hard to see something not happening—in this case, not dying—as a tangible reward. But it will be worth it when you realize one day that you are healthier (not to mention thinner) and feel so much better because your food intake is more nutritious.

Once you've adapted your life-style to these changes, you'll forget what the bad-health style of life was like. Changing your eating behavior for a healthy heart diet will make you feel better, look better, and function better. The rewards will be so great, you'll never want to go back to that old life-style.

STRATEGY

DOING IT—THE STEP-BY-STEP METHOD

Okay, Begin: Lose 1 Pound Per Week

Step 1: A suitable way to reduce high cholesterol or triglyceride levels (see Chapter Twelve for additional information) is to lose 1 pound a week. Suppose, during your caloric audit, you find that you eat about 2,200 calories per day, or about 15,400 each week. To lose 1 pound per week, you would need to eliminate 500 calories per day, or 3,500 per week.

This means you could either eat 1,700 calories per day or 11,900 calories per week to lose 1 pound. If your eating style is to eat more on weekends than during the week, you could eat 900 calories per day, Monday to Friday. This would leave you with 7,400 calories on Saturday and Sunday. It is unwise to consume less than 900 calories per day in an unsupervised situation.

Remember, the purpose of the initial calorie-counting is to give you some idea of how many calories you are eating each week.

Estimate the amount of calories cut on how much you now weigh. The average man eats about 12 calories per pound each day and the average woman, 11 calories per pound each day.

So, a 180-pound man would eat 2,160 calories a day, or 15,120 per week. If he eliminates 3,500 per week, he'll lose a pound by only consuming 11,620 per week, or about 1,600 per day. A 150-pound woman is taking in 1,650 calories a day at that weight. For her to reduce health risks through diet, she'd cut her caloric intake the same way.

Step 2: Now, look at *what* you're cutting. Since we are talking about making permanent changes in eating habits, examine your "audit" to see which foods are high in calories. If they have twice as many calories, which means twice as much fat, that's where to start. Learn to avoid or only rarely eat these food. *But, don't say you'll never eat them again.*

After all, it is necessary to be realistic when setting goals. What chance of success do you think you'd have with a plan that prohibited your favorite food? Not much. If, on the other hand, you know the amount of calories in pizza, you can save up on your calories that day and "spend" them on a pizza that night. Why not?

By learning the value of the foods you have eaten each day you can cut as many calories as you need. You should spend calories just the way you spend money. Ask yourself, is a 12-ounce steak worth spending 1,350 calories, or would you be just as happy with a 12-ounce filet of fish for 300 calories. If your cholesterol is down and you've been doing well lately, you may decide that the steak is okay for that time. The knowledge about calories lets *you* be in control—not some list or proscribed program.

If you approach weight reduction in this manner, you have begun actual behavior modification. When you have lost weight and kept it off because you have learned to eat different foods, then you've reduced your health risks from weight forever.

The second element of weight loss is exercise, which helps make calorie cutting less painful and is used to maintain a more healthful weight. Exercising in general and for caloric reduction specifically is covered on page 80 and in Chapter Twenty.

Step 3: Use the various charts that follow to determine what foods you want to eat, noting their caloric and nutritional value. Construct menus, using as much of your old eating style as you can. As we've said, if you can't live without pizza or cookies, substitute or sacrifice elsewhere to cut the calories necessary to lose pounds.

How to Use These Charts to Lose Weight

The charts on the following pages tell you about the value of the foods you eat. The charts give you three basic groups with calories per average serving included.

You can tell at a glance which foods are high in carbohydrates and protein, and low in calories. Use these charts to plan your needs. Involve the family.

The second chart gives you another strategic method of changing dietary habits. This chart tells you how to substitute basically low-value foods for better food. Using this chart, you can get rid of these foods while still satisfying your need for certain kinds of foods.

Step 4: Get enough food each day. One thing that anyone will tell you about changing what you eat is that it *can* get depressing. There is always the immediate reward that eating a big meal brings to make

CALORIE CHART: MEAT, POULTRY, FISH

CALORIES PER OUNCE (RAW WEIGHT)*

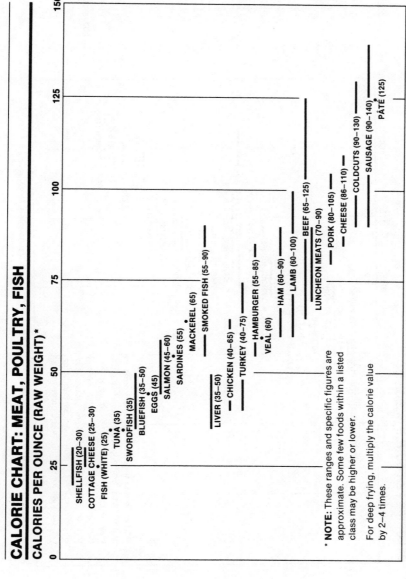

SHELLFISH (20–30)
COTTAGE CHEESE (25–30)
FISH (WHITE) (25)
TUNA (35)
SWORDFISH (35)
BLUEFISH (35–50)
EGGS (45)
SALMON (45–60)
SARDINES (55)
MACKEREL (65)
SMOKED FISH (55–90)
LIVER (35–50)
CHICKEN (40–65)
TURKEY (40–75)
HAMBURGER (55–85)
VEAL (60)
HAM (60–90)
LAMB (60–100)
BEEF (65–125)
LUNCHEON MEATS (70–90)
PORK (80–105)
CHEESE (86–110)
COLDCUTS (90–130)
SAUSAGE (90–140)
PÂTÉ (125)

0   25   50   75   100   125   150

* **NOTE:** These ranges and specific figures are approximate. Some few foods within a listed class may be higher or lower.

For deep frying, multiply the calorie value by 2–4 times.

© 1986 Lorraine Galante-Schwarz, Lawrence T. P. Stifler, Ph.D., Health Management Resources

CALORIE CHART: BAKED GOODS
CALORIES PER OUNCE (WEIGHT)*

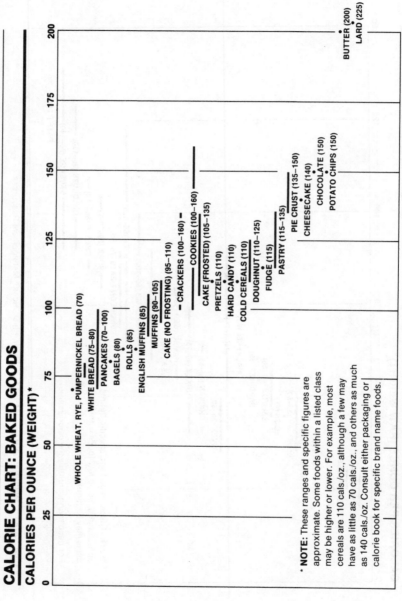

WHOLE WHEAT, RYE, PUMPERNICKEL BREAD (70)
WHITE BREAD (75–80)
PANCAKES (70–100)
BAGELS (80)
ROLLS (85)
ENGLISH MUFFINS (85)
MUFFINS (90–105)
CAKE (NO FROSTING) (95–110)
CRACKERS (100–160)
COOKIES (100–160)
CAKE (FROSTED) (105–135)
PRETZELS (110)
HARD CANDY (110)
COLD CEREALS (110)
DOUGHNUT (110–125)
FUDGE (115)
PASTRY (115–135)
PIE CRUST (135–150)
CHEESECAKE (140)
CHOCOLATE (150)
POTATO CHIPS (150)
BUTTER (200)
LARD (225)

* **NOTE:** These ranges and specific figures are approximate. Some foods within a listed class may be higher or lower. For example, most cereals are 110 cals./oz., although a few may have as little as 70 cals./oz. and others as much as 140 cals./oz. Consult either packaging or calorie book for specific brand name foods.

© 1986 Lorraine Galante-Schwarz, Lawrence T. P. Stifler, Ph.D., Health Management Resources

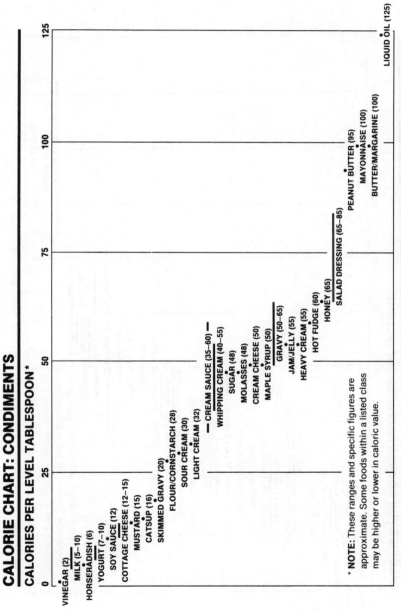

CALORIE CHART: CONDIMENTS
CALORIES PER LEVEL TABLESPOON *

0 — 25 — 50 — 75 — 100 — 125

- VINEGAR (2)
- MILK (5–10)
- HORSERADISH (6)
- YOGURT (7–10)
- SOY SAUCE (12)
- COTTAGE CHEESE (12–15)
- MUSTARD (15)
- CATSUP (16)
- SKIMMED GRAVY (20)
- FLOUR/CORNSTARCH (28)
- SOUR CREAM (30)
- LIGHT CREAM (32)
- CREAM SAUCE (35–60)
- WHIPPING CREAM (40–55)
- SUGAR (48)
- MOLASSES (48)
- CREAM CHEESE (50)
- MAPLE SYRUP (50)
- GRAVY (50–65)
- JAM/JELLY (55)
- HEAVY CREAM (55)
- HOT FUDGE (60)
- HONEY (65)
- SALAD DRESSING (65–85)
- PEANUT BUTTER (95)
- MAYONNAISE (100)
- BUTTER/MARGARINE (100)
- LIQUID OIL (125)

* NOTE: These ranges and specific figures are approximate. Some foods within a listed class may be higher or lower in caloric value.

© 1986 Lorraine Galante-Schwarz, Lawrence T. P. Stifler, Ph.D., Health Management Resources

CALORIE CHART: PREPARED FOODS
CALORIES PER 8 OUNCE PREPARED CUP (VOLUME) *

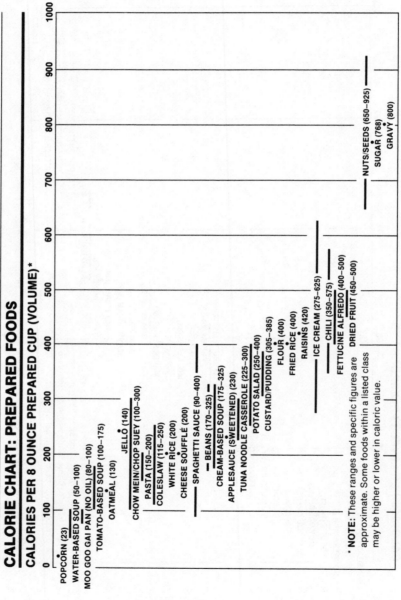

POPCORN (23)
WATER-BASED SOUP (50–100)
MOO GOO GAI PAN (NO OIL) (80–100)
TOMATO-BASED SOUP (100–175)
OATMEAL (130)
JELLO (140)
CHOW MEIN/CHOP SUEY (100–300)
PASTA (150–200)
COLESLAW (115–250)
WHITE RICE (200)
CHEESE SOUFFLÉ (200)
SPAGHETTI SAUCE (90–400)
BEANS (170–325)
CREAM-BASED SOUP (175–325)
APPLESAUCE (SWEETENED) (230)
TUNA NOODLE CASSEROLE (225–300)
POTATO SALAD (250–400)
CUSTARD/PUDDING (305–385)
FLOUR (400)
FRIED RICE (400)
RAISINS (420)
ICE CREAM (275–625)
CHILI (350–575)
FETTUCINE ALFREDO (400–500)
DRIED FRUIT (450–500)
NUTS/SEEDS (650–925)
SUGAR (768)
GRAVY (800)

* **NOTE:** These ranges and specific figures are approximate. Some foods within a listed class may be higher or lower in caloric value.

© 1986 Lorraine Galante-Schwarz, Lawrence T. P. Stifler, Ph.D., Health Management Resources

CALORIE CHARTS: FRUITS AND VEGETABLES

CALORIES PER OUNCE (WEIGHT/EDIBLE PARTS ONLY) CALORIES PER 8 OUNCE CUP (VOLUME)

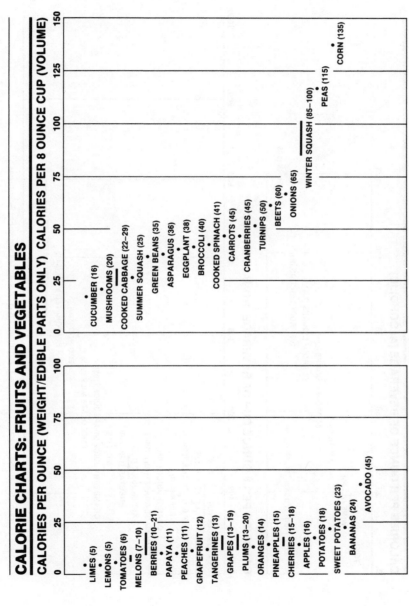

LIMES (5)
LEMONS (5)
TOMATOES (6)
MELONS (7–10)
BERRIES (10–21)
PAPAYA (11)
PEACHES (11)
GRAPEFRUIT (12)
TANGERINES (13)
GRAPES (13–19)
PLUMS (13–20)
ORANGES (14)
PINEAPPLES (15)
CHERRIES (15–18)
APPLES (16)
POTATOES (18)
SWEET POTATOES (23)
BANANAS (24)
AVOCADO (45)

CUCUMBER (16)
MUSHROOMS (20)
COOKED CABBAGE (22–29)
SUMMER SQUASH (25)
GREEN BEANS (35)
ASPARAGUS (36)
EGGPLANT (38)
BROCCOLI (40)
COOKED SPINACH (41)
CARROTS (45)
CRANBERRIES (45)
TURNIPS (50)
BEETS (60)
ONIONS (65)
WINTER SQUASH (85–100)
PEAS (115)
CORN (135)

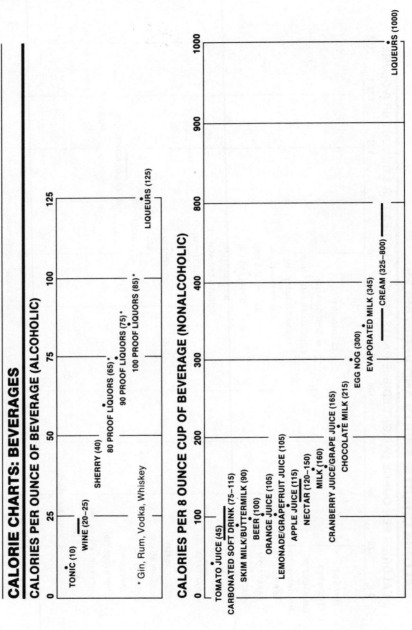

CALORIE CHARTS: BEVERAGES

CALORIES PER OUNCE OF BEVERAGE (ALCOHOLIC)

0   25   50   75   100   125

TONIC (10)
WINE (20–25)
SHERRY (40)
80 PROOF LIQUORS (65) *
90 PROOF LIQUORS (75) *
100 PROOF LIQUORS (85) *
LIQUEURS (125)

* Gin, Rum, Vodka, Whiskey

CALORIES PER 8 OUNCE CUP OF BEVERAGE (NONALCOHOLIC)

0   100   200   300   400   800   900   1000

TOMATO JUICE (45)
CARBONATED SOFT DRINK (75–115)
SKIM MILK/BUTTERMILK (90)
BEER (100)
ORANGE JUICE (105)
LEMONADE/GRAPEFRUIT JUICE (105)
APPLE JUICE (115)
NECTAR (120–150)
MILK (160)
CRANBERRY JUICE/GRAPE JUICE (165)
CHOCOLATE MILK (215)
EGG NOG (300)
EVAPORATED MILK (345)
CREAM (325–800)
LIQUEURS (1000)

you feel better. But for someone who has poor eating behavior, there is hidden harm.

For example, we know that protein-enriched foods are "good." But most Americans get twice as much protein as they need to maintain a healthy life-style. We also think that we have to have lots of red meat—you get protein, and after all, "the meat and potatoes" diet made America great, right?

Well, that's another myth. A complete vegetarian diet could give you all the daily protein you need. So, when you cut back on meat, you won't lose the protein you need. There are plenty of nutritious, nonmeat, high-protein foods.

Therefore, when planning any change, make sure that you don't starve yourself. You should not try to lose pounds overnight. *Your goal is to try to change the way you eat and how you think about food, so plan satisfying meals that curb your hunger.*

Stop for a moment and examine what we mean by "hunger." We have all experienced the gurgling stomach and lightheadedness that remind us to eat. In America, however, we treat hunger as a medical emergency to be alleviated immediately.

We have heard people say—routinely—that they are "starving." When we ride down the highway and the kids say, "I'm hungry," it's cause for an immediate pit stop to prevent acute malnutrition that might occur at that instant.

"I'm starving" is an exaggerated term in the United States for failure to eat at a usual time. You might find that the best way for you to lose weight is to completely eliminate a meal such as lunch. You *will* be hungry. You will not starve to death. The mildly unpleasant symptoms of delayed eating are easily ignored until they disappear. Soon you won't even notice them.

We've all seen the cartoons of dieters staring forlornly at a large, empty plate with a single radish on it. This is a myth; it is not how people lose weight. It's how people *don't* lose weight, but, instead, give up from frustration.

Here are some specific strategies to follow when constructing your new menus. Here is some vital information to learn and adopt as part of your dietary behavior:

GETTING ENOUGH PROTEIN

You don't have to sacrifice protein when you cut down on meat. There are plenty of nonmeat foodstuffs (pasta, legumes) that will give you all the protein you need, and with much less fat and calories. You can eat a very nutritious (and delicious) limited meat diet that will help you to lose weight and keep it off. Finally, we're not saying that you *have* to cut out meat altogether and become vegetarians. What we want you to do is:

DIETARY STRATEGY

1. Learn which foods are especially high in fat, oil, and cholesterol.
2. Cut down on these foods and use the suggested substitutes.
3. Get to the point where you can put together a healthy diet that meets your taste needs and *stick to it*.

TRIMMING THE FAT OUT OF YOUR DIET

Meat

Beef, pork, lamb, duck, and goose are especially high in fat. Organ meats (liver, kidney, brain) are very high in cholesterol. If you absolutely insist on eating these kinds of meat at your main meal (you should not eat them at lunch), keep it down to once or twice a week, with small portions. A slice of meat 4 inches wide, 4 inches long, and ½ inch thick weighs about 4 ounces. An average hamburger patty is 3 ounces.

As substitutes for beef, pork, and lamb, you can use chicken, turkey, lean veal, and fish. These foods have less fat and oil than the red meat group. This is important for the kind of diet we're seeking, because some fats and oils seem to raise cholesterol levels.

Avoid or Cut Down	Substitute
Beef, pork, ham, bacon, lamb, organ meats (liver, kidney, brain), sausages, hot dogs, and lunch meats.	Chicken, turkey, lean veal, fish, pasta, and beans.

Dairy Products

Milk products are another rich source of protein. Unfortunately, they are also loaded with fats. Whole milk, butter, cream, ice cream, and whole milk cheese all have a high butterfat content, and should be avoided as regular sources of calories. If you drink milk, make sure it's low-fat milk. Skim milk is the best of all (it just takes some getting used to). Also, cottage cheese and yogurt made from skim milk are good, safe protein sources.

What about eggs? They're great sources of protein, but the yolks are chock-full of cholesterol. So get rid of the yolks and eat the whites —that's where most of the protein is anyway. If you feel you must eat eggs that look yellow, buy egg substitutes that have artificial yolks made from corn oil. In any case, limit your egg intake to *two* per week.

How about baked desserts and pastries? Sad but true, most of these delicious goodies are full of animal fat and cholesterol (from shortening, cream, eggs, and butter). You don't have to write them off completely, but you can't live on them either. To sum up:

Avoid	Substitute
Whole milk, butter, light and heavy cream, half-and-half, sour cream, ice cream, whipped cream, cheese made from whole milk, egg yolks, and *pastries made from any of the above.*	Skim milk, yogurt, and cottage cheese made from skim milk, skim milk cheese, egg whites or whole eggs with artificial yolks.

Complex Carbohydrates

In the average American diet, most of the energy supplied comes from fats and carbohydrates. If you cut down on the amount of fat you take in, you have to boost carbohydrate intake in order to supply your body with the energy it needs. But here's where the matter gets tricky; we have to choose between "simple" and "complex" carbohydrates. *Simple carbohydrates* give you a quick rise in blood sugar that instantly cuts the hunger pangs, but they cannot sustain those blood sugar levels, and your appetite soon returns—which is no bargain for anyone trying to eat less. In other words, the simple carbohydrates give you quick energy (calories), but are digested too rapidly to satisfy

AVOID	SUBSTITUTE
Sugar, alcohol, soft drinks, sweets (candy and desserts), honey, and syrup.	Vegetables, fruits, potatoes,★ rice, grains, whole wheat bread, and pasta.

★ Surprise! A baked potato, contrary to popular opinion, is not fattening. It becomes a caloric disaster when you start loading on the butter, sour cream, and gravy. Likewise, pasta isn't fattening unless it's eaten with meat or cream sauces.

your appetite. In contrast, *complex carbohydrates,* such as vegetables, fruits, grains, and cereals, are digested slowly enough to provide nutrients over a long period of time. This is what we're looking for in our better heart diet.

Fiber

Some of the complex carbohydrates give you a fringe benefit—they're high in fiber, which is in short supply in the average American diet. Dietary fiber is basically the parts of plants that we cannot digest. It is found in vegetables like celery, lettuce, and corn, as well as in whole grains, cereals, and bran.

Fiber is apparently important in slowing down the digestion of carbohydrates and in keeping cholesterol from being reabsorbed into intestinal fluids. Although it has not been absolutely proven, fiber may also help in preventing cancer of the large intestine.

Salt and High Blood Pressure

The main problem with salt in our better heart diet is that excess sodium (a chemical in salt) may raise blood pressure in some people. For people with normal blood pressure, the slight rise caused by sodium isn't a problem. But for people with high blood pressure, sodium intake should be reduced to see if it helps bring blood pressure down.

STRATEGY

REDUCING SODIUM INTAKE

One of the difficulties in reducing our sodium intake is that it is in just about everything we eat: "Hidden" sodium accounts for as much

AVOID	SUBSTITUTE
Table salt, potato chips, corn chips, pretzels and other salted snacks, salted nuts, ketchup, pickles, and pickled foods.	Lemon juice, wine vinegar, garlic, spices, onion, radishes and other crunchy vegetables such as celery, carrots, and water chestnuts.

as 50 percent of our sodium intake. It's in processed foods, spices, sauces, pickled foods, and soft drinks. That's why it's necessary to read the labels on food packages—you can't always tell from taste alone. And while you can't completely avoid taking in sodium, you can cut down on the major sources and still get more than your body possibly needs.

Step 5: Here's another step to take—learn to shop right. Don't go to the supermarket when you're hungry—eat first. This is because you'll naturally want to buy items that are high in sugar and provide an instant reward. Also, make a very specific shopping list before you go. If you are focused when shopping, then you'll spend less time in the market wandering down tempting aisles.

Here are some specific things to learn about food shopping:

STRATEGY

SHOPPING FOR THE RIGHT FOODS

If you're absolutely dead-set on buying beef, purchase only the "good" or "standard" grades; the "choice" or "prime" cuts actually have more fat in the tissue, which is why they are more tender. Avoid meat that is heavily marbled with fat, and buy only pieces that are well trimmed. When you buy ground beef, make sure it is marked lean or extra lean.

When you get around to the dairy counter, reach for the low-fat milk, cheeses partially made with skimmed milk (such as farmer cheese), and yogurt made with skim milk. If you're determined to buy eggs, look for egg substitutes that contain the natural white portion but have vegetable oil substituted for the yolk. You can do most of the things with these eggs that you can with regular eggs: scramble them, make omelets, and use them in recipes. You just can't fry them sunny-side-up.

Now let's move on to the vegetable and fruit section: buy whatever you like. Make sure you pick up lots of lettuce, celery, carrots, cucumber, and tomatoes. These will be important for your snacks and salads. For main dishes, buy squash, eggplant, and potatoes.

A quick pass through the cereal section will take us past a wide assortment of breakfast choices. Whole wheat or rice cereals, as well as oatmeal, supply goodly amounts of protein. But read the labels carefully—some breakfast foods have more calories than others.

On your way out, pick up some pita (Syrian) bread or whole wheat enriched bread (read the label!). Avoid egg bread, cheese bread, or biscuits cooked with eggs and whole milk. Pass the pastry counter and turn your head. All the cakes, cookies, pastries, rolls, and doughnuts prepared commercially are made with natural eggs, whole milk, animal shortening, and butterfat—all of which, as you know, are rich in saturated fats and calories.

A final thought as you wait in line at the checkout counter: The racks of candy bars have been strategically placed there in case you can't wait to get home and open your food. Don't get trapped into such impulse buying. Chocolate has a very high saturated fat content and should be avoided in any form. Nonchocolate candies are no better, given the amounts of sugar they contain.

Step 6: What about eating meals? Both eating at home or eating in restaurants present potential pitfalls for the life-style-changing dieter. You may be part of a family whose dining requirements are such that you have to eat at a certain time. It could be early, leaving you hungry later on. It could be later, so you'll get the urge to "nosh" before dinner.

Eating out presents the kinds of problems that eating at home does, without the potential for change. Often people don't have a choice about eating out. It may be a business decision or it may be a social event you're invited to attend.

Here are some tips for cooking at home and dining out:

STRATEGY

PREPARING YOUR FOOD

Now that you've gone out and bought all kinds of healthy food, we have to spend a few moments talking about the best ways to prepare it. If you take your vegetables and sauté them in saturated oil, you really haven't gained a whole lot in terms of keeping your calories and cholesterol down. Before you start cooking, take a look at your supply of pots and pans. Do they have nonstick surfaces? If not, think about purchasing a set; nonstick surfaces allow you to cook without butter, margarine, or oil. You can purchase nonstick pots and pans fairly inexpensively at discount stores.

HOW TO COOK

Let's go back to that food you just bought, starting with the meats. Roasting, baking, and broiling are more likely to remove excess fat from meat than frying, braising, or stewing. Whatever you do, you should trim all the fat you can away from the meat before cooking it. Also, use a rack that allows the fat to drain away during cooking. Meat with a high content of saturated fat (red meat, organ meat, etcetera) should not be deep-fried; the crust just captures the fat that would ordinarily drain out. Meat with lower amounts of saturated fats (chicken or fish) can be deep-fried, as long as you use vegetable oil rather than animal fat. (Remember, though, deep frying doubles the calories because the oil gets absorbed into the food!)

Lean meat tends to be less tender than meat with high fat content. You can overcome this problem by braising, stewing, or tenderizing it. Low cooking temperatures and longer cooking will also make lean meat more tender. Finally, remember to remove all the fat from meat juices before using them to make gravy. Chill the meat sauces and remove the solidified fat.

What about sauces, garnishes, and dressings? Just avoid using cream, butter, or meat drippings. Whenever possible, use fresh vegetables, wine and spirits, meat broth, or cheese made with partially skimmed milk. Corn oil and safflower oil should always be used as substitutes when a recipe calls for animal fat.

When sautéing vegetables, you'll find that you really don't need any oil at all. Water will do. In fact, vegetables contain so much water that you can actually begin to sauté them dry—once the heat builds up, the water will quickly come out and keep everything from burning. Start off with medium heat, increasing it gradually until the vegetables are soft.

When a recipe calls for eggs, you can use either eggs with substitute yolks or just the egg whites. The yolks are included in recipes because they help hold the whole mixture together. An easy way to get along with egg whites alone is to remember that two egg whites are about equal to one whole egg. So, for every whole egg that's called for in a recipe, use two egg whites. For thickening, use flour or egg whites instead of oil. When cream is called for, use yogurt.

A final note about cooking: watch the salt. Even though a recipe might call for some table salt, you can do without it. Cultivate a taste for unsalted foods.

DINING OUT

You can go a long way toward controlling the fat content of food in your own kitchen. But what about when you go out to eat? A few simple rules will help keep you on course:

1. Whenever possible, avoid restaurants that feature fried foods. You should also avoid places that are heavy on pizza, cheese dishes, and combination dishes such as stews and casseroles.
2. Pick out restaurants that offer roasted, baked, or broiled entrees. Choose seafood, chicken, turkey, fish, and veal as often as you can.
3. Avoid sauces, gravies, and dressings made with cream, sour cream, butter, or cheese. You can, however, use lemon, wine vinegar, or low-cal dressings (you can always bring packets of low-cal dressings with you when you eat out).
4. Order vegetables prepared without butter, sauce, or margarine.
5. Avoid biscuits, rich pastries, cakes, cookies, pies, puddings, and ice cream. Instead, order plain bread and rolls, unfrosted angel food cake, fruit gelatin, or sherbet.

When eating out, here are some tips to help you eat a healthy and delicious meal.

French Restaurants

Try: An artichoke for an appetizer. It will take you at least 20 minutes to eat it and you'll only get 150 to 200 calories (if you go easy on the vinaigrette dressing and avoid the hollandaise); mussels vinaigrette (less than 100 calories); rack of lamb or fish (rack of lamb is better than lamb chops, since it is trimmed of fat before roasting; eat fish that is poached or served with plain sauces). Have fresh fruit for dessert.

Avoid: Anything prepared remoulade (which means with a mayonnaise dressing); onion soup made with cheese and bread; vichyssoise and other cream-based soups.

Chinese Restaurants

Try: Chinese spareribs (which are very lean and could make a main course); plain rice (only 100 calories per half cup); whole steamed fish in black bean or ginger sauce.

Avoid: Anything fried (including egg rolls, shrimp, rice, or noodles); ask that your meal be prepared without MSG, salt, or sugar.

Steakhouses

Try: Shrimp cocktail (double it for a main course); broiled shrimp; if you must eat prime sirloin, go easy (remember, even a small, 2 x 3 inches, 1-inch-thick piece has 350 calories and plenty of fat).

Avoid: French fries and onion rings (instead order the plain baked potato *lightly* seasoned, hold the sour cream and bacon).

Italian Restaurants

Try: Antipasto as a main course; pasta with a vegetable sauce; anything piccata-style (sautéed plain with lemon); for dessert try zabaglione (200 calories per serving).

Avoid: Garlic bread; meat sauces; foods prepared parmigiana-style.

Mexican Restaurants

Try: Plain corn tortillas with chili sauce for nibbling; tostada with vegetables.

Avoid: Tacos; enchiladas; corn chips.

Japanese Restaurants

Try: Sushi; sashimi; steamed fish.

Avoid: Tempura.

Seafood Restaurants

Try: Baked, poached, or broiled plain fish; go easy on shellfish (although they aren't as bad as once thought, they are high in cholesterol); pepper and lemon seasonings.

Avoid: Anything deep-fried or dipped in batter; tarter sauce; butter.

Salad Bar Restaurants

Try: Raw vegetables; dark green vegetables; vinaigrette or lemon dressing.

Avoid: Canned or pickled foods (beans, beets, etcetera); high-fat, creamy dressings; bacon bits; olives; pickles.

STRATEGY

EXERCISE AND YOUR HEART

The Benefits of Exercise

Exercise is beneficial to your heart for a number of reasons. First, it helps bring your weight down by burning off calories and reducing your appetite. It also helps in controlling blood pressure levels, which, as you know, is a very important factor in keeping your heart healthy. Also, regular exercise makes you feel better and look better, and also helps you to get more enjoyment out of your favorite activities. Finally, although scientists do not know exactly how exercise might protect you from heart attacks, it is well known that people who exercise suffer less heart disease than those who lead inactive lives.

Before going any further, we should spend a few moments to talk about the kind of exercise we're interested in. In terms of a healthy heart, *continuous* activities that use large muscle groups for more than

15 or 20 minutes are best. Walking and jogging are excellent examples. Of course, using the steps instead of an elevator, doing gardening, or moving furniture around are also exercise, because they require muscle work and energy. As far as your heart is concerned, however, these kinds of activities aren't very useful; they involve brief spurts of energy, which do not have the same beneficial effects as rhythmic, continuous exercise. (Nevertheless, the more you use your body, the more calories you burn—so it is worthwhile to park farther away than normal, to use the stairs instead of the elevator, and to devise other similar strategies.) Sudden exertions like lifting or pushing heavy objects around can also wrench a muscle, causing you pain and discomfort. Continuous exercise, when properly performed, gradually tones muscles so there is much less chance of straining or pulling. Finally, we're not looking at exercise as a way to develop huge muscles—that's not the goal. The rhythmic endurance exercise we recommend will build your stamina, redistribute your weight, tone flabby tissue, and improve your cardiovascular fitness.

So get into your shoes and start walking—the time investment you make in a regular exercise program will certainly be small compared to the tremendous benefits you'll soon reap!

How Much Should You Exercise?

If you've been inactive for a long time, it is very important not to go beyond your limitations. If there is any question about the safety of your plan, your doctor may want to do an exercise test. Here are a few good rules of thumb that will help you figure out if you're pushing yourself too hard. First, when you exercise and are still able to talk while doing so, you're within your limits. Second, if you can do an activity for an hour and still feel that you could do it for *another* hour, then you're still within your limits.

Benefits of Exercise

1. It builds your stamina so you can get more enjoyment from the activities you like doing.
2. It helps control blood pressure.
3. It keeps weight down.
4. It burns calories.
5. It reduces your appetite.
6. It tones muscles and gets rid of flab.

Finding Your Limitations	Starting a Walking Program
Rule #1. If you're breathing hard but still able to talk during your exercise, then you're within your limits. *Rule #2.* If you can do an activity for an hour and still feel you can go on for another hour, you're within your limits.	1. Begin your walk slowly, then work up to 100–130 steps per minute. 2. Walk for at least 30 minutes. An hour is even better. 3. Walk continuously—don't stop to chat.

Unless you're jogging or running, you should start your exercise program by walking briskly. If you have a watch, count how many steps you do in a minute; a brisk pace would be 100 to 130 steps per minute. For the first five minutes of each walk, start off slower, then gradually pick up the pace until you are walking briskly. Try not to break your stride; one of the biggest problems with walking is the tendency to stop and talk with friends. Remember, good exercise is *continuous*.

If you decide upon walking as your exercise program, each walk should be at least thirty minutes, although an hour would be better. In any event, establish a level that you're comfortable with, and work up from there. The same, of course, holds true with jogging or any other activity—never push beyond your limit.

How Often Should You Exercise?

The key to a good exercise program is *regularity*. It's far better to exercise moderately several times a week than to work out until you're exhausted once a week or once a month. An occasional strenuous workout can, in fact, be very dangerous. For those of you who are starting off with a walking program after a long period of inactivity, plan to walk at least three to four times a week.

How Often Should You Walk?
Regularity is the name of the game. If you are going to do a walking program, you should walk 3 to 4 times a week, for at least 30 minutes per walk.

Increase Gradually

Take it easy. If you've been out of shape for a while, pushing yourself to exhaustion can be very dangerous. Each time you increase your level, stay there for 2 or 3 weeks. Only advance comfortably.

If you are accustomed to playing doubles tennis, you should only play singles tennis for 10 or 15 minutes. If you are accustomed to running 1 mile, you should only run an extra quarter of a mile, and whenever you increase your distance you should not increase your speed at the same time. Try increasing your speed later. When you can cover a mile in 13 minutes then try to cover the same distance in 12 minutes. Once you can run 3 miles in 30 minutes, there's no medical reason you should ever try to do more.

How Should You Increase Your Activity Levels?

Gradually! The first time you increase your physical activity, you should do only a little more than you are accustomed to doing. If you are accustomed to walking, you should increase the time and speed until you can cover one or two miles four or five times a week. Whenever you do increase the level of your activity you should stay at the next level for two or three weeks. If the new amount of exercise tires you, it's too much and you should drop back to a more comfortable level. Eventually you will reach some level that you need not ever exceed. When you can eventually walk two miles three or four times a week, you will maintain a high level of physical fitness. (See the following box if you run or play tennis and want to increase.)

Symptoms to Watch For During Exercise

With any exercise program, there are certain symptoms and warnings that you should pay attention to, especially if you've been inactive for a long time and don't really know your limits yet.

1. *Chest Pain:* If you feel chest pain that starts during an exercise and stops when you end the activity, you should hold off on the exercise until you see a doctor. Chest pains that last for only a few seconds are usually not important—but that is for your doctor to determine.

2. *Difficulty in Breathing:* When you exercise, it is normal for the breathing rate to increase. The thing to watch for is a feeling of having to strain to get air into your lungs. If you do experience this kind of

difficulty in breathing when you exercise, stop the activity immediately and see your doctor before continuing with your exercise program.

3. *Unusual Heartbeat:* If your heart feels like it is beating too fast, beating irregularly, or pounding too hard when you exercise, you should check with your doctor before continuing with the program. Unusual heart sensations, such as very fast or irregular beats, are sometimes caused by taking too many stimulants, such as coffee, tea, or cola. Alcohol can also cause unusual heart sensations.

4. *Ankle Swelling:* Ankle swelling is caused by too much fluid being held in the body. If your ankles are bothering you and your weight has shot up more than 4 or 5 pounds in a few days, your body may be building up excess fluid. This is a problem that your doctor can correct. In the meantime, you should hold off on exercising. This can be a serious symptom and should *never* be ignored.

5. *Faintness:* If you feel faint during an activity, you should either stop the exercise or go at it a bit more easily. Don't push yourself to the point of exhaustion.

6. *Fatigue:* Feeling really tired after a day of exercise is usually due to the fact that your body has been inactive and isn't used to a workout. So, if you're tired the day after your exercise, there's usually no cause for alarm—in fact, it's even to be expected. If you find yourself so tired after exercising that you're uncomfortable, you should reduce the activity until you gain the strength needed to do it. It's not really surprising that some tiredness and weariness will be part of the picture until you're in shape.

Exercise Symptoms That Should Be Checked by Your Doctor
1. Chest pains
2. Difficulty in breathing
3. Unusual heartbeat
4. Ankle swelling with rapid weight gain

Warning Signs to Take It a Bit Easier
1. Faintness while exercising
2. Extreme fatigue after exercising

What Kinds of Exercise Should You Do?

Jogging, bicycling, swimming, and walking are the best cardiovascular exercises because they are continuous and rhythmic. Moreover, they allow you to build up the pace of activity and to control the amount of energy you have to expend. The chart at the end of the chapter shows you how much energy (in terms of calories) various types of exercise require.

In the final analysis, the best exercises for you are the ones that you *can* and *will* do. Whatever activity you choose, it should be convenient and pleasant. That's why at the minimum we want everyone in this program to walk three or four times a week. Once you've purchased a good pair of walking/running shoes, you're all set. You'll find that walking will build up your stamina, so that you'll be able to perform other activities with less effort. You'll also find that a regular walk is a good time to sort out your thoughts and feelings. If you're planning on walking before (or to) work, it might be a good way to get mentally ready for the day and think about any plans you've made. If you walk after work, it can be a good way to unwind from the day and resolve any problems that you had.

What Kinds of Precautions Should You Take?

1. *Take It Slow:* If you're out of shape, you should begin a program *slowly* to allow the muscles and joints of the body to become accustomed to increased activity. Overdoing the amount of activity in the first few sessions may cause you to become discouraged because of painful, sore muscles and joints. A beginner should take a few weeks if necessary to build up to his or her goal. If the program is to be four miles of walking each day, then a good start would be a mile or two at the beginning, with a gradual increase in speed and distance.

2. *Warm Up Slowly and Cool Down Gradually:* Take four or five minutes at the start of each exercise session to stretch muscles and bend joints before they are worked vigorously. Simple calisthenics, running in place, and short periods of running alternating with walking are good ways to loosen up before strenuous exercise. Toward the end of each exercise session, slow down your speed, decrease the intensity of your exertions, and end up by walking for five or ten minutes before you stop altogether. When you shower, use water with a lukewarm

temperature. Do not shower with steaming hot water and do not take a steam bath after strenuous exercise. Very hot temperatures enlarge skin blood vessels; after vigorous exercise, this may cause you to faint.

3. *Exercise Under Comfortable Conditions:* Strenuous physical activity in extremes of hot or cold temperatures makes your heart work harder than during physical activity under comfortable conditions. Cold temperatures make breathing difficult and cause blood pressure to rise higher than usual. Hot temperatures make the heart work harder circulating blood through blood vessels in skin and sweat glands. High humidity makes it difficult to lose heat by sweating. If the temperature is very hot or very cold, reduce the intensity and duration of physical activity to half your usual amount. It's probably best to take the day off. If you insist on exercising when conditions are not right, you may do yourself more harm than good.

4. *Avoid Physical Activity on a Full Stomach:* Digestion and absorption of food require circulation of blood through the digestive organs, while exercise requires circulation of blood through the skeletal muscles. Even a normal heart can't supply enough blood for both, and the result may be tired muscles, severe cramps in your abdomen, and extra work for your heart. Do not exercise sooner than forty-five minutes after a full meal.

5. *Exercise Only When You Feel Well:* Many diseases, such as upper respiratory infections, influenza, and dysentery, reduce the capacity of your heart and muscles to do physical work. Some diseases even have the temporary effect of weakening your heart for a short period of time. When you exercise even though you don't feel well, you make your heart work more than usual. There is no way exercise can hasten your recovery from illness, and the extra work may actually do harm to your heart. Wait until you have completely recovered from any illness before you return to your program of regular physical activity. When you do start again, do so at a lower intensity of activity and for shorter periods of time than usual. Gradually work your way back. Consult your physician about any symptoms that last more than one or two days, and ask him or her whether you should restrict your activities.

6. *Use Proper Shoes and Clothing:* Your shoes should provide good support to your feet and ankles, good traction for your footing, and

---

Exercise Precautions

1. Increase slowly; don't push
2. Warm up slowly, cool down gradually
3. Don't exercise if it's below 40 degrees F or above 90 degrees F
4. Wait 45 minutes after eating before exercising
5. Don't exercise when you don't feel well
6. Wear proper shoes and clothing
7. Follow your exercise prescription
8. See your doctor regularly

---

good soles to absorb the force from your feet striking the ground. Your socks should be thick enough to absorb moisture without making your feet hot and uncomfortable. Your clothes should not be so tight as to hinder your breathing or your movements, and not so loose as to get in your way. In cool weather, dress warmly in clothing that will absorb moisture. In hot weather, wear clothing that will protect you from the sun and allow perspiration to evaporate.

7. *Special Instructions:* Be sure that you understand what intensity and duration of exercise your physician has prescribed for you. Do not exceed the amounts of exercise that have been recommended for you. The best plan is to proceed slowly and safely.

8. *Consult Your Physician Regularly:* Too often patients fail to consult a physician when they feel well; they think about their health only when they become ill. Your chances of maintaining good health are greatest when you obtain medical advice *before* you become ill. See your physician at least once a year and consult him or her whenever you do not feel well. If you should ever develop unusual symptoms while exercising, you should consult your physician immediately. If you can't contact your physician, you should go to the emergency room of the nearest hospital and ask for medical advice.

Beating the High Blood Pressure Odds

Hypertension Kills by Causing:
• Atherosclerosis
• Angina pectoris
• Heart attack
• Stroke

High blood pressure, or hypertension, has earned its reputation as "the silent killer." Nearly 40 million Americans have it, many without even being aware that they do. In America, no other chronic disease is diagnosed or treated by doctors more often than high blood pressure. Around the world, it is estimated that high blood pressure may be involved in the premature deaths of 100 million people every year.

Sadly, many of these deaths could have been prevented if the disease had been diagnosed and treated earlier. Unfortunately, although many people have been told that they have high blood pressure, they—for whatever reason—neglect to do anything about it.

Fortunately, modern medicine has made tremendous strides in the treatment and control of high blood pressure through the wise use of medications and other preventive measures. Millions of lives can be saved if hypertension is discovered and treated before it damages the body.

WHAT IS BLOOD PRESSURE?

Blood pressure refers to the force generated by your heart as it pumps blood through your blood vessels. As we discussed earlier, with every heartbeat, your heart exerts pressure into your blood vessels; this pressure is called "systolic." Another kind of blood pressure is exerted when the elastic walls of the blood vessels push back against the blood; this other pressure is called "diastolic." In short, systolic pressure occurs when the heart pumps, or pulses, blood through the blood vessels, and diastolic pressure occurs when the walls of the blood vessels push back against the blood. Simply stated, high blood pressure means that too much force is needed to circulate blood throughout your system.

HOW CAN YOU TELL IF YOU HAVE HIGH BLOOD PRESSURE?

High blood pressure is called "the silent killer" because, unlike many other conditions, it usually does not have any symptoms. Very few people visit the doctor complaining of high blood pressure. In fact, most people are surprised when—usually in the course of a routine physical examination—they are told they have it. Most of us think that the typical person with high blood pressure is the nervous, frantic type who's constantly facing one crisis after another. But that's not true. High blood pressure occurs indiscriminately among all temperaments and all types of people: blacks and whites, poor and rich alike are all subject to it.

The only way to assess accurately whether or not you have high blood pressure is through measurements taken by a sphygmomanometer, or sphyg (pronounced *sfig*) for short. The typical sphyg consists of an inflatable cuff, a gauge to measure pressure, and a stethoscope. Usually a doctor or nurse will wrap the cuff around your upper arm, then inflate the cuff until the pressure of the cuff stops the flow of blood through your arm. Gradually, the cuff is deflated, allowing blood to circulate again. When the blood begins to flow, a loud thumping noise can be heard through the stethoscope.

The pressure indicated on the gauge when the circulation is heard to resume is the systolic pressure. As the cuff continues to deflate, the sound of circulation becomes fainter, because the blood circulates more easily. At the exact moment that the thumping noise stops, the pressure indicated on the gauge is the diastolic pressure. These two readings—the systolic and the diastolic—are usually combined as "110 over 80" or "110/80" (the 110 figure represents 110 millimeters of systolic pressure, while the 80 figure refers to 80 millimeters of diastolic pressure).

UNDERSTANDING THE "NUMBERS GAME"

Doctors interpret these numbers—the systolic and diastolic measurements—in a manner similar to a Las Vegas bookie determining the point spread in a football game. Statistics have told physicians that an average 35-year-old person with mild to moderate high blood pressure can expect to live only to about 60, if the high blood pressure is not treated. With normal blood pressure, this same person could expect to live to age 76! Clearly, the person with untreated high blood pressure is playing against the odds.

Years of statistical analysis have helped to establish the following guidelines for understanding your blood pressure levels:

- Normal blood pressure varies from a systolic pressure of 100 to 140 over a diastolic pressure of 70 to 85.
- Mild high blood pressure ranges from a systolic pressure of 140 to 159 over a diastolic pressure of 85 to 104 (85–90 is borderline).
- Moderate high blood pressure varies from a systolic pressure of 160 to 179 over a diastolic pressure of 104 to 114.
- Severe high blood pressure ranges from a systolic pressure of 180 and higher over a diastolic pressure of 115 and higher.

Where do you fit in? If you don't know, *please* find out.

THE DANGERS OF HIGH BLOOD PRESSURE

High blood pressure can lead to many serious health risks, from kidney damage to strokes. Some of these health risks are fatal; others may significantly worsen the quality of your life. Here's how high blood pressure, left untreated, can lead to health risks which can take years away from you:

Early Warning Signs of Stroke

Many people hit by stroke are warned, usually months in advance, that a stroke is imminent. The warnings come in the form of temporary strokelike symptoms, called "trans-ischemic attacks," or TIAs. Too often, TIAs are dismissed as unimportant unless their victims are alerted to them. A TIA is caused by the temporary blockage of blood to part of the brain. Some signs are:

- Dizziness lasting for a few minutes without apparent reason, such as after a carnival ride
- Numbness in the arms or legs, again without apparent reason, such as a sharp blow or other obvious injury
- Tingling (pins-and-needles sensation) in the limbs
- Temporary slurring of speech

Source: *The Pill Book of High Blood Pressure* (New York: Bantam Books, 1985).

Strokes

In North America, more than 400,000 people suffer strokes each year. One study found that people with high blood pressure are *seven times* more likely to have a stroke than people with normal blood pressure.

High blood pressure may cause a stroke by forcing blood through blood vessels already weakened by years of high blood pressure. When the blood spills into the brain, millions of brain cells die because they are deprived of blood. Even a tiny stroke can damage the areas of the brain responsible for hand and arm movement, balance, speech, or memory. Also, untreated high blood pressure contributes to atherosclerosis (hardening of the arteries). This condition may ultimately block the flow of blood to the brain, resulting in a stroke.

Atherosclerosis (Hardening of the Arteries)

Atherosclerosis is the result of fatty deposits building up in the arteries. If thick enough, these deposits may reduce the flow of blood, or even shut it off completely, causing a stroke or heart attack. Angina pectoris—serious chest pain resulting from a restricted blood flow to the heart—is the main warning sign that your arteries may be blocked by atherosclerosis.

People who have high blood pressure develop atherosclerosis twenty years before people with normal blood pressure and have a 200 to 400 times greater chance of suffering a heart attack induced by atherosclerosis cutting off blood to the heart.

Congestive Heart Failure Warnings

Congestive heart failure frequently causes edema, the buildup of fluids throughout the body, most noticeably in the legs. Ankles become swollen, even without extensive walking. Edema is persistent; it does not go away even after resting a few hours. The buildup of fluids in the lungs is another sign of congestive heart failure. Some symptoms to watch out for are:

- Persistent swollen ankles. If you press your finger against your ankle, and the depressed area pushes back out immediately, it may be a sign of edema, especially if the swelling came on gradually (over a period of a few months).
- Severe, persistent coughing, sometimes waking you up in the middle of the night, without a cause you can identify (such as heavy smoking). May be a sign of fluid buildup in the lungs.
- Persistent shortness of breath without corresponding exercise.

If you experience any one of these symptoms, consult your doctor.

Source: *The Pill Book of High Blood Pressure* (New York: Bantam Books, 1985).

Congestive Heart Failure

Congestive heart failure occurs when the heart is not strong enough to pump blood against the pressure of the blood already filling the blood vessels. In short, this is the battle between the systolic pressure (the pressure exerted by the pumping heart) versus the diastolic pressure (the pressure from the blood vessels). As the heart struggles to pump against the high diastolic pressure, it gradually grows weaker and weaker until it can no longer pump blood with adequate pressure. Since the heart can no longer effectively circulate the blood, fluids—which were once carried away—now begin to collect in the lungs, veins, and other areas in the stomach or legs. The collection of fluids within the body is called edema. Pulmonary edema, or the collection of fluids in the lungs, can lead to death.

People with untreated high blood pressure are four to six times more likely than people with normal blood pressure to develop congestive heart failure.

KIDNEY DISEASE

High blood pressure is a leading cause of kidney disease—a disease that kills 60,000 Americans each year. As a result of high blood pressure, arteries which supply blood to the kidneys may be damaged by atherosclerosis and blocked. The failure of the blood to circulate freely in a kidney means that the kidney can no longer efficiently cleanse the blood of waste materials. Untreated high blood pressure may ultimately result in kidney failure.

Also, since the kidneys produce a blood-pressure-regulating hormone called renin, any restriction of blood flow to the kidneys adversely affects the body's system of blood pressure control.

THE FIGHT-OR-FLIGHT RESPONSE

Under normal, everyday circumstances your blood pressure seldom remains the same. Whether you are standing, walking, or running, your blood pressure rises to meet the challenge. Similarly, when you are resting, your blood pressure drops.

The fight-or-flight response refers to the physiological reactions your body undergoes when confronted with a dangerous situation. When the brain perceives danger, your heart beats faster, your muscles tense, and your blood pressure rises. Your body is preparing you to either stay and fight, or to flee from the threatening situation. Sometimes the dangerous situation is clearly physical, such as a chance encounter with a mugger; at other times, the dangerous situation is less clearly defined (an angry boss who yells at you). When the dangerous situation has passed, your blood pressure should return to normal.

Such blood pressure fluctuations are the result partly of changing levels of various hormones and other chemicals in your body, which instruct your heart to beat faster or to slow down.

Other chemical and electrical impulses tell your blood vessels to constrict so that blood will flow to your limbs and more blood will be available for your heart and vital organs.

These impulses are transmitted by hormones such as *epinephrine* and *norepinephrine*—which are made by the adrenal glands on top of your kidneys—and by *baroreceptors* (pressure-sensitive cells that are part of your central nervous system). Your kidneys also produce another substance, called renin, whenever your blood pressure drops. Renin stimulates the production of other hormones that tighten your blood vessels and raise your blood pressure.

Obviously, your body employs a very complicated system of automatic responses to regulate your blood pressure. A condition of abnormally high blood pressure can develop when just one step in this regulatory system goes haywire. Your blood pressure constantly runs at full speed, continually overworking your heart and blood vessels, no matter how nonthreatening your situation is.

WHAT CAUSES HIGH BLOOD PRESSURE?

There are two types of high blood pressure: *secondary hypertension* and *essential hypertension*.

Secondary hypertension affects only 3 to 5 percent of the people who have high blood pressure. This type of blood pressure has a distinct identifiable cause, and if this underlying condition is corrected, blood pressure usually returns to normal. Secondary hypertension is caused by conditions ranging from kidney ailments to blocked arteries to birth control pills. In many cases, secondary hypertension can be corrected by surgery, or simply by treating the original condition that precipitated the hypertension.

Essential hypertension affects 95 to 97 percent of all people who have high blood pressure. Because of the complex system your body uses to regulate hypertension, no one knows precisely what causes essential hypertension. While doctors do not know the exact cause of essential hypertension, they *do* know several factors that play an important role in high blood pressure. Many of these factors (also called "risk factors" since they increase the risk of your having high blood pressure) can be controlled by you.

HYPERTENSION RISK FACTORS

Heredity: Studies show that hypertension, like other physical traits, can be inherited. If one parent has high blood pressure, there is a good chance that one out of every four children will develop hypertension. And if both parents have high blood pressure, it is likely that half of their children will have it, too. This doesn't mean that children of parents who have been diagnosed as hypertensives, or who have suffered from one or another of the illnesses brought on by high blood pressure (e.g., heart disease, stroke, kidney disease) will automatically become hypertensives. There is a chance that you may never have high blood pressure, even if you have every risk factor for hypertension. However, if your family history indicates that you run the risk of developing high blood pressure, then you need to keep especially close tabs on your blood pressure. The earlier a diagnosis is made and treatment begins, the greater the chance against damage being done to your health.

Obesity: Being overweight means that you face a greater chance of developing high blood pressure. Excess weight means that your heart must work harder to circulate the blood throughout your body. While not everyone who is overweight has high blood pressure, there is still a strong statistical link between the two.

For adults, almost any weight gain—even if only a few pounds—tends to increase your blood pressure. And if you already have high blood pressure, any weight gain can be very dangerous.

However, losing weight—even if only a few pounds—will ease the burden on your heart and decrease your blood pressure.

Exercise: Lack of exercise contributes to your chances of having high blood pressure. Many studies comparing inactive people to those who exercise regularly have shown that exercise lowers blood pressure.

It is difficult to establish a direct link between exercise and lower blood pressure, since it is unclear whether it is the exercise, or the weight loss that usually accompanies exercise, that is responsible for the lower blood pressure.

Salt: Whether or not excessive salt leads to high blood pressure is a hotly debated subject within the medical profession. While there are experts on both sides of this issue, the scientific evidence, at this time, remains inconclusive.

Table salt, also known as sodium chloride, is a substance that consists of 50 percent sodium. Sodium helps the body retain fluid, and usually greater fluid levels lead to increased blood pressure.

But some studies have shown that there is little or no difference in hypertension rates between those who use little salt and those who consume significantly larger amounts.

Nevertheless, most doctors agree that reducing your salt intake certainly won't do you any harm, and may ultimately decrease your chance of having high blood pressure.

Calcium: Some new studies suggest that a diet deficient in calcium leads to hypertension. Some physicians advise their hypertensive patients to eat more calcium-rich foods. More studies are needed to establish a definite link between a lack of calcium and high blood pressure.

Stress: There is no doubt that any kind of stress, whether at work or at home, will raise your blood pressure. However, usually your blood pressure returns to normal when the stressful situation has passed. Most healthy people can stand repeated temporary exposure to stressful situations without developing high blood pressure. It is prolonged, virtually unrelenting stress that may lead to hypertension, especially if the stress is accompanied by a feeling of loss of control. The stress faced by telephone switchboard operators, who *must* answer call after call for eight hours a day, is potentially more troublesome than the stress an executive *might* face (the executive can simply tell a secretary to hold all calls). See Chapter Eight for more on this.

But not everyone who experiences constant stress develops high blood pressure. Your personality type may play an important role in determining whether or not you have high blood pressure. Those people who feel a constant sense of competitiveness and who are never satisfied with their accomplishments are classified as *Type A* personalities. Since they often view everyday events as emergencies, their heart rate and blood pressure may constantly be elevated. Type A personalities are especially prone to heart disease if they also have one or more of the other risk factors. (See Chapter Eight for more information.)

Type B personalities are more "laid back," less competitive and may be less likely to develop hypertension. (For more information on stress and Type A behavior, please turn to page 109.)

Race: High blood pressure is one reason why blacks have a shorter life expectancy than whites. A black American has a 50 percent greater chance of having hypertension than does a white American. Exactly why this happens is unknown. It may be because of heredity, or perhaps, since health care is not as easily obtained by blacks as it is by

Hypertension Won't Hurt You If:
• You take your medication exactly as prescribed • You have your blood pressure checked regularly • You keep your doctor up-to-date on side effects and work with your physician on the best possible means of treatment

whites, hypertension in blacks goes neglected until strokes and heart problems appear.

STRATEGY

BECOME A PATIENT

First, have your blood pressure checked on a regular basis. If you are told that you have high blood pressure, make an appointment to see your doctor *promptly*.

Realize that even though you don't feel any pain or discomfort now, it is extremely important, for your health and for your future, to get your blood pressure under control. Your doctor can diagnose the illness, prescribe the medications, suggest changes in your life-style, and warn you about the dangers of hypertension, but it is you, and you alone, that must take control of your future. You can do this by *becoming a patient*. Becoming a patient means taking your condition seriously: See your doctor on a regular basis and take any medication exactly as it is prescribed.

Your doctor may also suggest other life-style changes, such as losing 20 pounds, getting more exercise, trying to relax more often, and stopping smoking. In many cases, attempting all these changes, while also taking your medication, may be impossible. If you are hesitant to attempt these changes at once, ask your doctor what he or she recommends that you do *first*. Frequently, your doctor will suggest that you get your blood pressure under control by taking your medication. Once your blood pressure is under control, then you may feel capable of trying the other life-style changes.

Often, people leave the doctor's office after a diagnosis of high blood pressure determined to go on a diet, to start jogging the next morning, to stop smoking immediately, and to take their medication. Sometimes, after a few days, they fail to stop smoking. A couple of days later they go off their diet. And soon they stop taking their medication. They are ashamed to admit these failures to their doctor, so they neglect to go to their next appointment. And their high blood pressure continues to damage their bodies.

Only do one thing at a time when you enter treatment for high blood pressure. First take your medication and, with your physician, see that it's the right medicine and dosage for you. Then attempt life-style changes or other treatments.

If you try life-style changes and fail, don't give up; continue to take your medication and get your blood pressure under control. Admit to your doctor that you had problems maintaining the life-style changes, but continue to see your doctor on a regular basis. Perhaps at a later date, with your blood pressure under control, you may be able to lose weight or to stop smoking.

Other people find that their medication causes unpleasant side effects, such as nausea, vomiting, or headaches. These side effects may cause some people to stop taking medication and to blame the doctors for giving them a "bad" drug. If you experience a side effect while taking a medication, you should call your doctor *immediately*. Do not stop taking the medication until you have spoken with your doctor. Your doctor may change the medication or its dosage strength to lessen any discomfort caused by the side effects.

In most cases, taking your medication will allow you to control your hypertension, thereby minimizing a potentially life-threatening health risk.

STRATEGY

TAKING—AND UNDERSTANDING—YOUR MEDICATION

Medicine has provided physicians with a wide array of high blood pressure medications (also known as antihypertensives). Today, your doctor can prescribe safer and more effective antihypertensive medications than at any other time in history.

Some antihypertensive medications work by decreasing the amount of fluids in the blood. Other antihypertensives work by affecting the central nervous system, which ultimately controls everything that the heart and blood vessels do. Still other drugs work by loosening the muscles that tighten the blood vessels, thereby making it easier for blood to flow.

Most doctors treat hypertension with one of two possible drug treatment plans.

Course A: In some cases, the doctor may first attempt to control your hypertension by prescribing a diuretic, which reduces the fluid content in the blood. If the diuretic alone does not sufficiently control your blood pressure, the doctor may decide to add a beta blocker to slow your heartbeat. If these drugs still do not lower your blood pressure, your doctor may decide to add a vasodilator, which opens your blood vessels wider. And if all three of these drugs fail to lower your blood pressure satisfactorily, your doctor may prescribe yet another drug, which acts directly on your central nervous system.

Course B: Some hypertensive people respond better to a treatment plan that begins with a beta blocker. A diuretic may still be added if treatment with the beta blocker alone does not prove satisfactory. If this strategy does not work, your doctor may add a vasodilator or a drug that works directly on the central nervous system.

These treatment plans—either Course A or Course B—are referred to as "Stepped-Care Drug Treatment." This method begins with the mildest form of drug therapy and proceeds to more powerful medications, if necessary. The following diagram may help you to understand Stepped-Care Drug Treatment better. In my practice, 90 percent of hypertensive patients achieve blood pressure control with one or more medications.

Stepped-Care Drug Treatment

COURSE A	COURSE B
Step One	*Step One*
Begin with Diuretic	Begin with Beta Blocker
Step Two	*Step Two*
Add Beta Blocker	Add Diuretic
Step Three	
Add Drug to Dilate Blood Vessels (Vasodilator)	
Step Four	
Add Drug Acting on Nervous System or Angiotensin System	

You should understand that your doctor may need several weeks or longer to find the type and dosage strength of medication that works best for you. In the meantime, you should always inform your doctor of any side effects you may be experiencing.

GENERAL INFORMATION ABOUT THE DIFFERENT DRUG CLASSES

Diuretics: Diuretics have been a standard first-line treatment for high blood pressure since the 1950s.

They help to reduce blood pressure by reducing the amount of fluid in the blood. Less fluid makes it easier for the heart to pump blood, thereby reducing your blood pressure. Diuretics cause the excess fluid to be eliminated from the body with urine. The result is the most common side effect of diuretics: an increase in the frequency of urination and in the volume of urine.

Diuretics used as antihypertensives are divided into different groups according to their chemical structure and to where they act in the kidneys.

Thiazide and *thiazidelike diuretics* (e.g., hydrochlorothiazide, chlorothiazide, chlorthalidone) are frequently used to begin the drug treatment program. If these fail to control your blood pressure, more powerful loop diuretics (e.g., furosemide, bumetanide) may be tried.

The major drawback to these diuretics is their potential for causing electrolyte and mineral imbalances (such as potassium loss) in your body. If you are taking diuretics, pay close attention to possible signs of electrolyte imbalance (potassium loss): dryness of the mouth; thirst; weakness; lethargy; drowsiness; muscle pains or cramps; gout; decreased frequency of urination and amount of urine; abnormal heart rate; nausea; and vomiting.

If potassium loss affects you, your doctor may prescribe a potassium-sparing diuretic (e.g., spironolactone, triamterene) to counteract potassium loss. Your doctor may also prescribe a diuretic combination medication (where one ingredient is a diuretic and the other ingredient counteracts potassium loss). Or your doctor may suggest you take a potassium supplement or eat a diet rich in potassium (e.g., bananas, citrus fruits).

Beta Blockers: Beta blockers may be prescribed as the first drug treatment for hypertension, or after other drugs have failed to lower blood pressure. They may be prescribed alone or in combination with other drugs.

Exactly how beta blockers (e.g., atenolol, nadolol, metaprolol, pindolol, propranolol hydrochloride, timolol maleate) work is not known. It appears they lower blood pressure by blocking the effect of stimulants on the "beta" receptors found in the heart and in some blood vessels. Beta blockers reduce blood pressure by slowing the heartbeat, reducing the amount of blood pumped by the heart, dilating some major blood vessels, and by blocking the effects of naturally occurring stimulants.

Vasodilators: In general, vasodilators (e.g., hydralazine hydrochloride, minoxidil) are prescribed after other antihypertensives have failed to lower blood pressure. These drugs reduce blood pressure by relaxing the muscles responsible for tightening blood vessels, thus lowering your blood pressure by making it easier for your heart to pump blood.

Antiadrenergic Agents: Antiadrenergic agents (e.g., clonidine hydrochloride, prazosin, methyldopa, guanadrel, guanethidine) inhibit nervous reactions (called adrenergic reactions) believed to be responsible for increased blood pressure. In general, these drugs are prescribed after other antihypertensives have failed to lower blood pressure. They are frequently used in combination with other drugs to lower your blood pressure.

Rauwolfia-derivative drugs (reserpine, alseroxylon) are also considered antiadrenergic agents. These drugs appear to make it easier for your heart to pump blood by their ability to decrease resistance within the blood vessels. Like other antiadrenergic agents, these drugs are usually prescribed after other medications have failed to lower blood pressure.

ACE Inhibitors: The drug captopril is the first member of a new class of drugs (ACE inhibitors) that affect the production of hormones and enzymes involved in the regulation of blood pressure. Captopril lowers blood pressure quickly, usually within a half hour to an hour after taking the medicine. However, this drug can cause serious side effects and is usually prescribed only after other antihypertensive medications have failed to lower blood pressure.

STRATEGY

TRADITIONAL NONDRUG TREATMENTS

Your doctor may suggest that, in addition to medication, you try nondrug treatments to help control your blood pressure. In some cases these treatments, such as exercise, diet alterations, and stress reduction, may be so successful that your doctor may ultimately suggest that you stop taking medication.

Weight Loss: As stated earlier in this chapter, a weight loss of just a few pounds will usually result in a lowering of your blood pressure. For more information on how to lose weight successfully, see Chapters Six and Twelve.

Exercise: Promotes both weight loss and lower blood pressure. It is important to consult with your doctor before beginning an exercise program. For more information on exercise strategies, see Chapters Six and Twenty.

Stress: Gaining the ability to cope with stress is another means of controlling your blood pressure. For more information on stress and Type A behavior, see Chapter Eight.

Smoking: Your doctor may also suggest that you stop smoking. While a direct connection has not been made between smoking and hypertension, it is clear that people who smoke *and* also have hypertension are sixteen times more likely to suffer a stroke than people with high blood pressure who *do not* smoke! Clearly, smoking and hypertension together are a deadly combination. For more information on ways to stop smoking, see Chapter Nine.

STRATEGY

ALTERNATIVE TREATMENTS

While most doctors prefer to treat hypertension with drugs and/or traditional therapies such as weight loss and exercise, nontraditional methods are available for those who wish to try alternative means of controlling their blood pressure. Most of the more successful alternative methods of treating hypertension deal with handling stress. As stated earlier in this chapter, most people respond to stressful situations with a "fight or flight" response, which automatically raises blood pressure. If you can be taught to confront a stressful situation by relaxing instead, your blood pressure is less likely to rise dangerously.

Before embarking on an alternative treatment plan, you should be aware that many alternative methods require a major commitment of time—a commitment that not every well-intentioned person can afford. You should also note that none of the alternative methods have been as consistently successful as prudent drug treatment plans.

Yoga: Of the many nontraditional treatments for hypertension, yoga may provide the greatest benefits. Some of the systems taught by yogis enable people to relax, sometimes to the point where their blood pressure decreases. Yoga exercises should always be learned under the guidance of a trained, qualified instructor.

Zen Buddhism: In a manner similar to yoga, the meditation techniques of Zen Buddhism may allow you to lower your blood pressure.

Transcendental Meditation (TM): Transcendental Meditation, or TM, can be learned by anyone in just a few hours. The individual gets in a comfortable position, breathes regularly, closes his or her eyes, and repeats a word or "mantra" (at first aloud, then silently). A mantra is usually a word-sound from the Sanskrit language.

Progressive Muscle Relaxation (PMR): PMR attempts to control stress through the rhythmic tightening and relaxing of certain muscles. PMR can be done in virtually any position, and at any time.

Biofeedback: Biofeedback uses an electrical device that lets a subject know when a desired physical or mental state has been reached. For example, a buzzer might go off whenever the subject's blood pressure goes above a predetermined level. The subject then tries various relaxation techniques in an attempt to keep blood pressure below this level.

Beating the Stress Odds

STRESS—FUEL FOR OUR FIRE

Many people feel that stress is responsible for all their problems. If they could only relieve their stress, their lives would be simple, uncomplicated, and smooth sailing. But the role stress plays in our lives is not that simple. While it is true that stress is a major risk factor for heart disease and a variety of other syndromes affecting several organ systems, stress can also be used to your advantage.

Stress can be the fire that fuels the daily furnace of production. In its broadest definition, stress is merely anything that evokes a response from you. It does not have a positive or negative connotation; stress can be good or bad.

The cardiovascular system, for example, doesn't know whether the home team is winning or losing, it only responds to your excitement by speeding up and pumping harder. It's the inappropriately exaggerated response to stimuli (called "stressors") that may be harmful, unless you learn how to cope with these episodes of overresponse. As long as you can keep your responses appropriate, stress seems to do no harm and actually protects us from hazards in our environment.

It is when you lose control of these responses that stress seems most destructive. Only common usage makes the word "stress" all bad.

Although we adopt that common usage in this chapter, remember it's not the stress but how you respond that's important.

Stress may also be a risk factor whose time—scientifically—has finally come.

A lot of us grew up with the cliché "It's all in your head" used when we had symptoms like a headache or stomachache with no clear-cut cause. "Psychosomatic illness" has been replaced by new terms: "stressors," "hot reactors," "burnouts." These new terms are partly a result of our greater understanding of the mechanism of stress —both good and bad. We have learned that the brain (which is "in your head") can react to stress and cause diseases as serious and life-threatening as a bad heart.

The brain controls glandular systems that release hormones, which, in turn, control our central nervous system. As we've been able to examine how this mechanism works a little better, we have concluded that many diseases can be affected by the brain. And you can reduce your risk of these diseases by control of your mind and reduction of the stress situations you encounter.

WHAT IS STRESS?

The word "stress" has become quite commonplace in our vocabulary: We're constantly told that we live in a high-stress society in which the pace of life is too fast and the pressures are too great. And we're told that we must learn to cope with stress, because it has harmful effects on our bodies. But what does "stress" really mean?

According to the scientist who pioneered stress research, Hans Selye, it's "the rate of wear and tear within the body." Others have referred to stress as "a metaphor for life."

In science, "stress" is neither good nor bad; it's just the body's way of reacting to events in the environment.

Stress becomes harmful when the rate or response is unnecessarily great, a situation that can be called "negative stress." With negative stress, the body is continually in an "alarm state"—that is, it is tensed and geared up for an emergency (this will be discussed in detail later in the chapter). But negative stress is only one side of the coin. "Positive stress," such as a challenge that you readily accept and enjoy, can actually enhance your life and spur you on to greater productivity and satisfaction. The secret is in remaining in control of that stress.

Unfortunately, though, the stress most people encounter is of the negative kind, and keeping it under control is not a simple matter. This chapter will teach you various ways to do just that. You can experiment with each approach to stress control and see which one works best for you.

WHAT ARE STRESSORS?

It's a little easier to describe stressful situations than to give a narrow definition of stress, especially since stress is different for every single person. For some people, a promotion to a new job is a stressful situation. For others, it's impending surgery. For some, stress occurs during a move from one home to another or simply from a new assignment at work. These events are what we call "stressors."

Stressors are, according to Selye, anything that results in a response by the body. Their effect is an exaggerated physical response such as causing a rise in blood pressure or stomach acid production or even too much "awareness" leading to insomnia.

They are positive when you are in control of life and stressors are responded to as challenges. When you encounter a problem and your response is exaggerated, then you are a "hot reactor."

Stressful situations have one common element: They all create a change in the order or balance of your life. Stress occurs when your established life-style—that routine you've worked so hard to establish—is upset or even threatened. Stress occurs when you must react to an event by altering what you normally do or modify your surroundings.

Obviously, one person's stressful situation may be another person's norm. Often your reaction will be a knot in the stomach or a pounding heart. Your blood pressure will rise, your breathing will increase, you may begin to sweat. This is known as a *stress reaction*. When your normal coping mechanisms are overloaded, you experience a physiologic stress reaction which occurs in various stages.

Recently, scientists have clarified the stages of the stress reaction. Their research has changed our minds about the effects of stress on our bodies.

WHAT HAPPENS DURING STRESS?

It could be said that your first response to a stressor is to "turn on." In effect, you get those old juices flowing. Your pulse rate quickens. As more blood pumps in your body, more oxygen is supplied to your muscles. Your blood sugar level increases, your pupils dilate, digestion decreases, while perspiration increases. In short, your brain perceives a stressor by setting off a chain reaction to prepare you for a violent response called "fight or flight." This response should be evoked only when your brain perceives a dangerous stressor.

The emotions you encounter stimulate a part of the brain called the hypothalamus, which acts on the autonomic nervous system and the pituitary glands to cause hormones such as adrenaline, beta endorphins, thyroxine, insulin, cortisone, and others to prepare the body for defense. Also during stress:

- The adrenal gland releases chemicals called "catecholomines" (adrenaline) that in turn cause the kidneys and blood vessels to raise blood pressure, and the heart pumps more blood.
- The brain releases "beta endorphins" that can affect your perception of pain.
- Corticosteroids, another naturally occurring substance, can also be released by the adrenal glands during stress. They affect the body's immune response to infection, leaving us open to disease.

It's obvious that what we have is a mind-body linkup. So while the stress reaction "may be all in your head," the effect is clearly physiological.

As these reactions occur during stress, the body does adapt. The bodily functions adjust, and the anxiety you feel from these changes will diminish as you take steps to cope or if the stressor disappears. *But,* the body can only take so much of a stress reaction. So if you don't adapt or cope, the body's supply of adaptive energy diminishes. If the body is stressed enough without relief, these physiological changes can do permanent harm. This is why stress is exhausting and why unrelieved stress can lead to disease, or early mortality.

DISEASES LINKED TO STRESS

Over 5 million people in the United States suffer from peptic ulcers, which may be related to an inability to control stress. Heart attacks and strokes are also linked to stress, although stress may not actually be a direct cause. Backaches, sexual problems, headaches, sleep disorders, nervousness and anxiety, skin problems, and even serious, clinical depression can be caused by stress.

Studies have linked the effects of stress on kidney disease, liver function, pancreatic production, bone marrow diseases, and stomach problems.

Other, more controversial research asserts that certain types of cancer can be linked to stress. Cancer risk factors such as cigarette smoking can also be increased by stress, according to these reports. Stress also affects our immune system, which helps fight cancer and infections.

Diabetics whose blood sugar control is vital have more complications from their disease when their emotions are out of control. Too, asthmatics are much worse off in stressful environments.

Researchers have also discovered another, very important aspect of the stress/disease link:

Failure to cope with stress hinders your body's natural abilities to fight off disease. Developing an ability to cope can actually help prevent disease. Several studies have revealed connections between the brain, the brain's ability to cope with stress, and the effect on the immune system. The breakdown of the immune system relates not only to the growth of cancerous tumors but also to debilitating allergies and the ability of the body actually to prevent cancer.

DETERMINING IF STRESS IS A PROBLEM FOR YOU

Over the past ten years, a number of researchers have proposed ways of identifying people who need to change the way they cope with stress. One of the most widely popularized systems is the concept of

---

It's not whether or not you have stress, but how you respond to those stressful events that creates the disease risk factor and affects its magnitude.

the Type A and Type B person, developed by Dr. Meyer Friedman and Dr. Ray Rosenman.

In short, the Type A person constantly feels a sense of time urgency and takes on more tasks than he can possibly handle. Type A personalities are also easily rattled and tend to look at all tasks as if they were being performed inside a pressure cooker.

In contrast, the Type B person goes along at a relaxed pace and doesn't feel that a constant "weight" is pushing on him. This isn't to say that Type Bs don't accomplish anything; their *attitude* is such that their work and responsibilities aren't sources of anxiety. The key, of course, is the word "attitude": with Type A behavior, even non-threatening, simple tasks can appear threatening and complex; the Type B can see the tasks for what they are and take them in stride.

There are studies that show that extreme Type A personalities have more cardiovascular disease than extreme Type Bs. The Type B outlook is clearly a healthier one, and may help to control problems such as high blood pressure and bodily aches. If you'd like to find out more about Type A and Type B behavior, read *Type A Behavior and Your Heart* by M. Friedman and R. H. Rosenman, which explains the concept in detail, and provides a self-test to help you determine which category you fall within. They have also recently released a newer book on the same subject, *Managing Type A Behavior,* which is a very helpful source of additional information for anyone concerned with this problem.

While the Type A/Type B distinction is useful, there are other ways of looking at how people handle stress. One is to simply ask yourself the following questions:

1. Is it hard for you to unwind during your free time?
2. Do you need a tranquilizer or a drink to relax?
3. If you're upset about something, do you find that your thoughts race through your mind at night so you can't sleep?
4. When you're tense or anxious, do you feel the need to eat or smoke?
5. Do you often get so worried that you have indigestion, diarrhea, or nausea?
6. Are there people or situations in your life that make you feel uptight just by thinking about them?
7. Do you feel that you're almost always racing against the clock?

If you answer yes to one or more of the above questions, then you ought to think about making some changes in your life-style. That may mean spending a good bit of time trying the following stress management approaches. But be assured that the payoffs will be well worth whatever time and energy you invest: You'll find it easier to relax and you'll sleep better. You may even find yourself getting more work done because you feel better.

COPING WITH STRESS

Your *Beat the Odds Health Profile* has identified several aspects of your life-style that cause stress-related risk factors in your life.

You may be reading this section of the book because you have been identified as a Type A personality, or you are at risk for some of the diseases we have mentioned. In addition, you may be generally unhappy and not coping too well in your daily life.

Here are some strategic moves you can make, remembering, of course, that simply reducing stress itself is an overall strategy for curbing risk for heart attack, stroke, high blood pressure, and other health problems.

STRATEGY

HOW TO HELP YOURSELF STOP TYPE A BEHAVIOR

Type As, as we discussed, are people who display very similar kinds of behavior. They walk, eat, and generally move fast. They never seem to have enough time and are often quite impatient. Type As hate to stand in line and aren't great in traffic jams either.

In short, Type As are aggressive, competitive, and frequently excessively hostile, angry, or irritable. But not every Type A person has every Type A characteristic. In some, certain aspects are more pronounced. Some Type As may not have the explosive speech patterns commonly found in this group, but they may be more likely to measure their success in terms of dollars or number of miles they jog than non-Type As.

When Type As are responding to certain challenges, the physical reactions they have are almost identical to the so-called stress reaction. Type A behavior has definitely been linked to heart attacks, and Type As also have more frequent second heart attacks.

Scientific research also shows that Type As have higher levels of cholesterol in their blood—perhaps because of that behavior. So, when stress is present in Type As and blood pressure is raised, the heart may not get enough oxygen because cholesterol buildup has narrowed their arteries. The result: risk of heart attack.

Changing Type A behavior requires some overall life-style changes. While entire books have been written on this subject, you can actually begin to change by taking just a few simple steps. Of course, recognizing that you are Type A is the most important step, but try these ideas, too:

1. Accept the fact that it's possible to be hard-working and successful without aggression and hostility.

   When you get angry for any reason, ask yourself: Am I too angry in relationship to what the event represents? *Awareness leads to change.*
2. Make a decision to set aside a certain amount of time each and every day for the rest of your life for relaxation. It is absolutely not necessary to work all of the time.
3. Recognize those situations that lead to Type A responses in your behavior and reorganize your life to avoid them. For example, if you hate to wait in line at the bank, don't go at lunchtime when the lines are longest. Start on your way to work earlier if being late disturbs you.
4. Look into a time management course or book to help you use your time better.
5. Start an exercise program that you enjoy.

Hand in hand with modifying Type A behavior is general behavioral change as a self-help strategy for stress reduction.

Change your behavior for yourself. If you think that you're doing someone else a favor when you change a bad habit—stopping smoking, for example—you aren't really making a change.

LEARNING TO COPE—A BASIC PLAN

It sounds simple, but coping may lie at the root of stress reduction. Most of us learn to cope by example, from our family, friends, and also our own experiences. Most of us are better equipped for coping than we may think.

Developing your coping strategies is a prime task.

One way to cope is called "adaptive coping" by experts, but what it really means is that you learn to use your "successful" methods over again. You should know from previous experience which coping methods you've used before actually work (like getting good advice, meeting a problem head-on, or taking a break when things get too strenuous). These methods of coping are almost always better because they result in the resolution of a stressful situation. Adaptive coping is not accomplished by ducking a problem.

If you haven't reduced your stress when you cope with a situation, then you've coped badly. This is called "maladaptive coping." We all have done this, whether it's going on an eating or drinking binge, avoiding responsibility for a mistake, or refusing to cope at all. This leads to chronic stress overload, which leads right to the doctor's office.

In many cases, maladaptive coping is manifested in Type A behavior. This is often because we don't want to be decisive in our actions. While you may "want" to cope properly, you haven't learned really good ways to cope.

This is an especially important self-help strategy. Seek new ways of coping well by reviewing how you handled each prior stressful situation. If you relieved the source of stress—not just temporarily removed it—then you have learned a successful tactic. But if you haven't, then you may need more help.

Coping well is always one of the best strategies that you can use to turn stress to your advantage. If you've learned ways of meeting those stress-filled challenges and not letting them get to you, you can avoid stress-related risks. Coping well is certainly part of beating the odds. It's not easy. It takes some thought and even some practice.

All of us, every day, do little things that become automatic behavior. For example, the person who doesn't like to fly or travel but has no choice works out methods of coping. I know one person who has to go to California every six months on business. He hates being cooped up on a plane. So, he takes his headset, at least two magazines, a book, and at least an hour of work with him.

By the time he's gone through all of the "activities" he's brought with him, he's crossed the country. Our friend has faced the fact that his "thing" about travel had to be coped with rather than avoided. He probably will never remove the phobia he's developed, but he will function.

SOME MORE STRATEGIES FOR COPING WITH STRESS

Adjusting Your Attitudes and Goals: The way you react to situations largely depends on your attitudes and personal philosophy. You can cut out a large source of minor irritants by just deciding that you're not going to let little things bug you—especially when they're beyond your control.

For instance, when you run into a long line at the gas station, movie theater, or restaurant, you can either fume or just think to yourself, Well, it's worth waiting for, and there's nothing I can do to shorten the line. So I'll just be patient—getting mad won't help. Or if you get stuck in a traffic jam, you can sit and stew in anger or you can say to yourself, There's nothing I can do about this, so I'll just sit calmly and use this "dead time" to plan out the rest of the day's activities.

What about your goals—do you regularly set and reset career and personal goals? Are they realistic? Striving for something that is essentially unattainable can be a great source of stress and anxiety. You might be struggling to obtain something that you can never really get. Or you might be counting on a great stroke of luck coming your way and changing your life. In the meantime, you could be avoiding certain problems at home or at work while waiting for the good fortune to knock on your front door.

Try writing down your immediate and long-term goals. Read them aloud. Do they really seem reasonable and attainable? If not, write down ways that you can make your goals more realistic. You might also want to read your goals to another household member—does he or she think that you can achieve your goals? If not, talk about why

STRATEGY: ADJUSTING ATTITUDES

Decide that you're not going to let unimportant things or situations beyond your control bother you.
Set realistic immediate and long-term goals.
See if others find your goals realistic and attainable.

STRATEGY: REHEARSING FOR STRESS

Rehearse future meetings and encounters in your mind's eye. Play things out as you would like them to happen.

your goals might be unrealistic for you. Then talk about how you might modify and bring them within your reach.

Rehearsing Stressful Situations in Your Mind: Your ability to create images in your mind's eye can be a powerful tool. If you're faced with an unpleasant or stressful task, like a meeting with your boss or a confrontation in your household, you might rehearse the scene in your mind. Imagine what it will be like. Imagine what you want to say and what you want to happen. This kind of mental rehearsal can give you a kind of script to follow. It can also help you to organize your thoughts and identify what you want. Getting some inkling about the unknown can be very helpful in reducing your anxiety. Even if the actual encounter goes very differently from the scene in your mind's eye, you'll be much more relaxed about it.

Avoiding Stressful Situations: There is absolutely nothing wrong with avoiding certain situations that are very stressful to you. If rush-hour traffic jams make you uptight, plan not to be driving in rush-hour traffic, or take a detour that might be a bit longer but will skirt the main roads. If you know that a certain kind of party or get-together is going to be downright unpleasant, pass up the invitation and don't go. If there's a particular kind of meeting that you don't like attending, see if one of your coworkers can go for you. In many situations, of course, you have to be present and a representative won't do. Still, when possible, consider avoidance as an honorable way of reducing your stress level.

Managing Your Time: There are only so many usable hours in a day. And you don't want them completely jammed up with appointments or things to do. Managing time is probably the hardest stress-reducing

STRATEGY: AVOIDING STRESS

When possible, avoid situations that are likely to make you tense or uptight . . . think of ways to reduce your stress.

task for most people. As a result, poor time management is a major cause of stress. The feeling of not having enough time to do everything you have to, let alone time to relax, can make a person tense and anxious. When this goes on day after day, life can become a losing race against the clock.

There are several things you can do to manage your time better. First, plan to fill up only one-half of your time with meetings, appointments, and things to do. You'll be surprised at how quickly unexpected things will pop up and fill out the rest of your day. Don't pack more and more into less and less time.

Second, use a planning book or calendar. The most helpful kind are those that show a whole month at a time; you can keep tabs on how each week is shaping up, and whether or not you're overloading yourself. Give yourself enough time between appointments and meetings to relax. Always look at your planning book or calendar before committing yourself to a definite appointment time. And take into account how long it will take you to get to and from appointments, as well as how long it will take you to readjust your train of thought.

This applies to recreational as well as business appointments. For instance, you might have a softball game scheduled on a Saturday afternoon and dinner out with some friends Saturday evening. Before you make a definite time for dinner, think about how long it will actually take you to get back from the baseball field. How far away is the field? How heavy is the traffic likely to be? Remember, whenever you feel as if you're in a time crunch, you're likely to be tense and anxious. Avoid this with good, realistic planning.

Organizing Work and Setting Priorities: The other aspect of time management is organization. Make daily lists of things that you have to get done. Think about what things are related and might be done together, so as to save time and energy. For instance, if you have to meet with two people who are located at the other end of the town, see if you can arrange for the meetings to be on the same morning or afternoon, so that you're not running back and forth. If you have errands to run, think about which ones could be done at the same time. You can save a lot of wear and tear on your feet and tires by grouping related activities together. The better you plan out the order and timing of things to be done, the less likely you're going to feel exhausted from racing against the clock.

Finally, there is the matter of meeting deadlines and setting priori-

STRATEGY: TIME MANAGEMENT

1. Plan to fill up only *half* of your time with scheduled events.
2. Use a planner or calendar, and don't schedule the whole day full of back-to-back tasks.
3. Make lists of things you have to do every day.
4. If you're on a deadline, allow time for unexpected problems.
5. Rank tasks by importance.

ties. In general, people whose jobs require them to meet deadlines constantly are under a good deal of stress. Even if they're perfectly capable of meeting the deadlines, unexpected events can always take place, so that a routine deadline becomes a battle against time.

Some veterans of constant deadline pressure go by what is known as Murphy's Law: Whatever can possibly go wrong *will* go wrong. To safeguard against this, allow extra time for unexpected problems; don't assume that everything—or anything, for that matter—will necessarily go smoothly.

Deadline planning also requires establishing priorities. If your time is limited and there's a lot to do, make a list of what tasks have to be done first. Rank each task by importance. If it looks like it will be impossible to get everything done in one day, work on only those tasks that need to be done immediately. Remember, you can't always do everything that you want to do or think you should be doing. That's why it is important to list everything you have to do and think about how you'll spend your energy.

COPING DIRECTLY WITH STRESS: RELAXATION

As you know when you are feeling stress, your body is geared up for "fight or flight": your heart rate, breathing rate, and blood pressure increase so that your muscles have plenty of blood, your muscles are tensed and ready for action, your blood is shunted away from your stomach and intestines and sent to your muscles, and your body chemistry changes so that you have plenty of energy. This is a survival state that pulls you through emergency situations that require quick reflexes and a spurt of strength. Unfortunately, it's also the way our bodies respond to many situations that don't actually lead to a fight-or-flight. So, when we think about an unpleasant event or feel rushed or aggravated, our bodies get ready for action. Many people live in a continuous fight-or-flight state, and suffer the harmful effects of alarm responses such as elevated blood pressure. This is why learning to live with stress is an important part of controlling blood pressure.

One way to deal with stress is to reverse some of the bodily effects of the fight-or-flight state. For instance, when your body is revved up for an emergency, the temperature in your hands will drop slightly, because blood is being diverted to your muscles. So, if you can relax and make your hands feel warm, you'll redivert your blood flow back to your extremities and bring yourself down from the "emergency ready" state to a calmer, healthier state. You can do this by practicing the "deep muscle relaxation" technique described at the end of this chapter. Once you're skilled at muscle relaxation, you should start practicing "mind relaxation" twice a day.

After practicing muscle and mind relaxation twice a day, fifteen minutes per session, you'll find that your ability to unwind from the fight-or-flight state will become almost automatic. But that takes time. You must start off in nonstressful situations. If your week is hectic, then delay practicing until a time when things are calm. Once you get better at relaxing, you can start using your new skills in stressful situations.

For instance, instead of having a cup of coffee on your break, find a quiet place and do some muscle relaxation. You can also start budgeting in some time to do muscle and mind relaxation before meetings and appointments, if they are a source of stress to you.

When you've really mastered muscle and mind relaxation to your satisfaction, you can go on to "instant relaxation," also described at the end of this chapter. This will enable you to give yourself a "relaxing calm" just about whenever you need it. Again, when you're starting out, only practice when you aren't feeling stress; you are much more likely to succeed and work up to instant relaxation if you learn the techniques when you're calm. Then you can apply them to stressful situations.

REDUCING STRESS: USING ASSERTIVENESS

Your personal relationships with family, friends, and coworkers can be great sources of joy in your life. They can also be great sources of stress when they aren't going harmoniously. It is normal to experience occasional friction even with close friends and loved ones. The way a

STRATEGY: ASSERTIVENESS

1. Helps you vent your anger in a constructive way.
2. Means communicating your needs, goals, and opinions in a forceful yet nondomineering way.
3. Should only be attempted when you are calm and relaxed.

person responds to that friction can make all the difference in terms of stress.

For example, everyone experiences anger throughout the course of the week. Many people keep their anger bottled up, until they are ready to explode. Then some minor incident happens, and they let loose, expelling a lot of rage at someone who doesn't deserve it. Pent-up anger can also lead to a host of bodily aches and pains, as well as other stress symptoms.

At the other extreme, some people automatically blow up whenever they feel hurt or wronged. This kind of defensiveness is no better than holding it all in. The midpoint between the extremes is effective communication in which you assert your needs, goals, and opinions in a forceful but nonpushy or nonthreatening way. Don't try to deal with the other person until you're relaxed. Use the relaxation techniques mentioned earlier if you need to calm down. If the other person is too mad to talk to reasonably, then wait until he or she cools off. Remember, being assertive does not mean being domineering. You'll find an example below of how an assertive encounter might go.

You and a coworker have been given an assignment, and you feel as if your colleague has taken the easier part of the work. You could:

A. Blow up and scream at him
B. Think about what a lazy person he is, and stew about it

or

C. Collect yourself and say, "Let's look at this assignment. I feel that you have less to do than me. It would be fairer if we broke it down so that we both have to put in about the same amount of time. Let's work together to divide it up. Here's my idea for an equal division. I'd like you to take a look at it." (This, of course, is the kind of assertive response that we're encouraging.)

STRATEGY: DIVERSIONS

Hobbies, sports, and recreational activities are important in managing stress. They take your mind off your worries, and give you other outlets for your energy.

DIVERSIONS

Hobbies, crafts, and sports can greatly help you unwind and take your mind off your worries. These activities are also important in that they offer you alternative ways of spending your energy, and provide a chance to meet with other people. If you're involved with a certain craft or creative art, try to find clubs or organizations devoted to that activity. Contact with new people will help balance out your daily work pressures, and will give you a fresh perspective on your problems.

REDUCING STRESS WITH EXERCISE

Some stress researchers maintain that physical exercise is the best way to reduce stress. From a common-sense point of view, there is an apparent truth to that idea; we all know that a good walk, run, swim, or other sport is a great way to "blow off steam." But you don't have to wait until the pressures build up—a regular program of physical exercise will make it easier for you to respond to situations that are potentially stressful. Recent research suggests that vigorous physical activity actually activates our own natural internal tranquilizer (endorphins), confirming that good feeling we experience after exercise!

Read Chapters Six and Twenty for suggestions on exercise.

Deep Muscle Relaxation

1. Pick a time you can practice relaxation on a regular schedule. This should be a time when you will not be interrupted or feel hurried. Choose a time before meals or at least one hour after a meal.

2. Choose a quiet, warm, comfortable environment where you will not be interrupted. Sit in a comfortable chair where you can relax completely. Or, lie on your back on a pad or a couch with a low pillow under your head in a comfortable position. Close your eyes.

3. Begin by tensing and relaxing groups of muscles on your "dominant side" (right side for right-handed people and left side for left-handed people). Tense the muscles of your hand by clenching your fist for a second or two, then relax them and let your hand muscles go loose. Try to make your hand feel warm and heavy. Continue with the muscles of your forearm, then your upper arm, and finally your shoulder. Eventually your hand, arm, and shoulder should all feel relaxed, warm, and heavy. Wait for these feelings before continuing with other muscle groups.

4. Next, tense and relax the muscles of your foot and leg on your dominant side. Tense the muscles of your foot by curling your toes for a second or two, then relax them completely. Try to make your foot feel warm and heavy. Continue with the muscles of your calf and your thigh. Eventually your foot and leg should feel warm and heavy.

5. Then, tense and relax the muscles of your *other* hand, then your arm, and then your shoulder. When you have made these muscles relax completely, your hand, arm, and shoulder will feel warm and heavy. Continue with the muscles of your foot and leg on that side.

6. Next, relax the muscles of your hips, buttocks, and pelvis without tensing them first. Concentrate on creating a wave of relaxation that spreads over your body from your pelvis, to your stomach muscles, and into your chest. Make the muscles feel warm and heavy. When all these muscles are relaxed, your breathing will come more from your diaphragm and stomach than from your chest. Wait for this change in breathing pattern before continuing.

7. Finally, concentrate on feeling the wave of relaxation in the muscles of your back, neck, jaw, face, and scalp. Concentrate on relaxing the muscles of your eyes and forehead. The skin of your forehead should feel cool when all the muscles are relaxed.

8. Practice this exercise for 15 to 20 minutes twice each day. With practice you should be able to relax all your muscles within 2 or 3 minutes. Once you are able to relax completely you will not need to tense and relax separate groups of muscles. You will be able to relax completely without first tensing any muscles and without relaxing each muscle group separately. Until then, however, you must concentrate on each group of muscles in turn.

Mind Relaxation

1. Begin by relaxing completely using the deep muscle relaxation technique. You should be comfortable, your eyes closed, your arms and legs warm and heavy, your body relaxed, your breathing deep, slow and from your stomach, your back, neck, jaw, and face muscles relaxed, and your forehead cool.
2. Become aware of your slow natural breathing. Concentrate on each breath as you inhale and exhale.
3. Clear your mind of thoughts. If thoughts do pop up, try to stop them with commands to yourself such as "let go."
   Or, imagine a pleasant scene, such as a lake, a field, a mountain, or drifting white clouds in a blue sky. Concentrate on this scene to suppress active thoughts.
   Or, do some repetitive, monotonous mental task such as mental arithmetic or repeating a list of names. Use this monotonous mental task to replace active thought processes.
   Or, try softly repeating a word that has pleasant meanings, or a sound that has no meaning at all; this might help clear your mind of unwanted thoughts.
4. Eventually, you should achieve a state of complete mental relaxation without images, thoughts, sounds, or words in your mind.

Instant Relaxation

1. Practice deep muscle relaxation and mind relaxation twice daily until you can become completely relaxed, physically and mentally, within 1 or 2 minutes.
2. Instant relaxation should be practiced in addition to regular relaxation, until you can relax under almost any circumstances.
3. Sit or stand in a comfortable position.
4. Take a deep breath, count to 5 slowly, exhale slowly, and concentrate on relaxing all the muscles you're not using to hold your posture.
5. Clear your mind of thoughts and try to ignore your surroundings. Concentrate on pleasant thoughts, imagine pleasant surroundings, and slow your mind as much as you can. Use any specific commands to yourself that you have used successfully for mental relaxation, such as "let go."
6. Practice instant relaxation many times during the day. Eventually, you should be able to relax quickly and effectively, even under stressful conditions.

STRATEGY

GET SOME PROFESSIONAL HELP

Most of us can take care of simple medical issues—cuts, colds, headaches, burns, bruises—but *seeking professional help may also be an important self-help strategy*. However, one thing you never want to do as a self-help strategy is to undertake self-treatment with drugs. Some of the effects of stress on a body in poor health may be controlled by diet and over-the-counter medications such as sleeping preparations. But this is not a great idea. Despite the fact that we successfully diagnose and self-treat three out of four of our own medical problems, we may not be as successful with stress.

So stress reduction can also come from outside. Not all of us have the inner resources to cope alone, and not everyone can readily identify the sources of their stress. Some people are already suffering from debilitating health problems caused—unknowingly—by stress, so there's no reason *not* to seek help from others.

You may not realize that stress is your problem, but if you do know that you are not well for unexplained reasons, the subject should be discussed with your own family physician.

A good doctor should ask you how things are going in your life when he's examining you for symptoms of a variety of diseases. This is something that *you* should also bring up, even if your doctor is only giving you a physical examination.

In any event, you should seek professional help with stress if it has been identified as the source of your physical distress.

Professional help comes in a variety of forms, depending on the source of stress. Since family physicians in the United States treat over 90 percent of all medical problems, they are often integrally involved in the patient's life-style. Finding a good family practitioner who can give you counsel or a good referral for further treatment is crucial.

You can contact the American Academy of Family Practitioners (AAFP) to locate certified FPs in your area. AAFP headquarters is located at 1740 W. 92nd Street, Kansas City, Mo. 64114. Or contact the American Society of Internal Medicine, 101 Vermont Avenue, Washington, D.C. 20005.

Another word about self-help strategies. You, in the end, are totally responsible for your own care and for taking steps to deal with stress.

You don't have to deal with your problems alone, though, and there are self-help strategies that can involve other people.

While the rule of thumb is always to take a physical exam if you think your health is changing or may be affected by stress, you may also want to seek some sort of psychotherapy to help you cope better. There are many ways to go about this, including writing to your state medical association for recommended psychotherapists or your local mental health association. These professionals can also be referred by your local community services organization (such as the YMCA) or religious group.

STRATEGY

MAKE SOME ENVIRONMENTAL CHANGES

Stress in the workplace is most often cited as a source of professional and health crises. Some of this may stem from your own Type A behavior, but some may be directly related to the nature of your job. For example, the rates of high blood pressure among bus drivers are far greater than among the rest of the population.

Here are some specific strategies that you can use to reduce stress in your environment:

Step 1: Clearly identify the sources of your stress. Is it a physical reaction to the work environment? Does this call for a communication with your superior or a visit to the company physician? What will changing your work environment do to your standing in your job?

Step 2: As we indicated, you can determine different methods of travel that are less stressful, or at least reduce travel anxiety. If you can fly one way and come back on a train, perhaps that will reduce the stress of air travel somewhat.

Step 3: Redefine yourself. If your job or occupation is very stressful, then it may be the wrong place for you. Money cannot replace health! So, consider vocational counseling or a transfer to another department that would reduce your stress.

Step 4: Relocate yourself. It's possible that your long commute twice a day is the source of your stress. Try to change that part of your life.

It may be possible to live elsewhere, but you've just not considered it seriously. Balance the value of the place you live in against the value of your health.

Step 5: Many people don't consider their marital or other personal relationships as "environmental stressors," but they may be. As you try to identify your source of stress, this is a question to ask yourself: Is my marriage or my lover hurting me? If you aren't sure (or are sure) you need professional help, don't delay a minute in seeking it. You may not be able to devise a simple strategy for changing this kind of stress, since it involves one or more people. So be fair to others in attempting to cope with this sort of problem.

STRATEGY

SEEK SUPPORT GROUPS

Patient support groups are a new and rising phenomenon on the American health-care scene. A recent survey found over 1,100 such organizations, dealing with 270 conditions, in the Chicago area alone. One source claims that there are 15 million Americans who are members of some 500,000 patient groups. These groups concern themselves with everything from divorce, to bereavement, to trauma, to suicide, to agoraphobia. These groups are a way for people to survive in an often chaotic world.

In addition to local groups, there are national clearinghouses to help people find the right group for their particular problem. Many of these clearinghouses have developed regional networks.

Self-help groups are ideal places to find solutions to both your own stress and stress induced by family problems. One thing that can increase your stress—and create other problems, such as guilt—is the effect of a family member's chronic disease on you and the rest of your family.

Patient support organizations often devote much of their attention to helping out family members with financial problems, cutting red tape, solving practical problems like transportation or housing near a hospital, or offering medical referrals. They also offer support for those suffering from a disease. There's nothing quite as reassuring as having someone who's been through a traumatic event describe the details firsthand. Not only is such reassurance a large benefit of a patient support group, but they are often good sources of advice. People talking to people about their medications or their experiences at one medical facility or another can be very helpful and mitigate the stress that builds up during a serious medical event.

There is no national or local "stress reduction" foundation, and most patient support groups tend to be problem-oriented. But there are many other types of organizations that can help with stress reduction: exercise groups, organizations that give training in meditation or biofeedback, etcetera. Some of these charge a fee and others are run by nonprofit organizations.

There are also many adult education courses offered by community colleges, local school systems, and private organizations that might help eliminate some of the sources of stress in your life. For instance, if you are having some sort of professional difficulty that creates stress, then perhaps you can find a course to help you improve your skills. And, there are also courses that do deal with stress reduction techniques in the home or at work. Some of these courses might help you deal with other sources of stress, such as in your marriage or other parts of your personal life.

Beating the Smoking Odds

The best part about smoking is stopping. People who stop smoking feel better, have fewer colds, less absenteeism, healthier children, a cleaner environment, and live longer than their fellow smokers.

WHAT WE KNOW ABOUT SMOKING

It's almost impossible to justify smoking cigarettes, or using any tobacco product, at least from the point of view of a physician interested in reducing the odds of premature death. We can state categorically: *Smoking cigarettes is the foremost cause of preventable death in the United States today. This means that the more than 350,000 Americans who died due to the effects of cigarette smoking last year should still be alive. More people die in one year from smoking than died in WW I, Korea, and Vietnam together.*

Smoking makes no sense at all. Yet, despite information that smokers are smoking less, the number of smokers is still staggering. Although per capita smoking has declined, there are still, according to the federal government, 1.5 million more smokers in the United States today than there were ten years ago.

In 1964, Americans smoked 511 billion cigarettes; today the number is 593 billion. Although smoking defenders point out that this is less than the peak 640 billion reached in 1981, at the same time, consumption of smokeless tobacco products has soared from 95 million pounds in the 1970s to over 132 million pounds in this decade. The *direct* cost of cigarette smoking to our health-care bill is $16 billion per year! Indirect costs are $37 billion.

To put these appalling numbers in perspective is the fact that it means that 45 to 50 million American people still smoke and, what's worse, the fastest-growing segment of this market is teenage girls, followed by teenage boys. In all, there are 1 million new teen smokers a year! Since the length of time you smoke is a prime aspect of smoking risk, these teenagers are getting a head start on bad health.

Despite new programs set up by the government to warn people of the dangers of smoking, the effect has been minimal. A new law, the Smoking Prevention and Health Education Act, passed in 1984, was supposed to strengthen warnings on cigarettes. But the Office on Smoking and Health has only a $3.5 million funding budget. The government spends four times that amount to just *administer* the tobacco subsidy program for farmers!

CIGARETTE SMOKING—A MAJOR RISK FACTOR

Cigarette smoking is not just a bad habit, it is a life-threatening one as well. The more cigarettes you smoke, the more damage you can do to your heart, lungs, and blood vessels. Cigarette smoking is a major coronary risk factor, because it raises blood cholesterol levels, reduces your lung capacity, and may damage the inside of blood vessels. If you've never had a heart attack and you're 33 years old, then each cigarette you smoke could cost you about 23 minutes, in terms of living to 68 years of age, which is currently the average age to which we live. (You can figure this out by starting with the fact that a cigarette smoker lives eight years less than average.) If you smoke a pack a day, then:

- Each *day* you smoke could cost you about *8 hours* off your life
- 5½ minutes of life are lost for each cigarette smoked
- Each *week* you smoke could cost you about *2 days* off your life
- Each *month* you smoke could cost you about *8 days* off your life
- Each *year* you smoke could cost you about *3½ months* off your life

One major reason why cigarette smoking is so dangerous is because it is actually more addictive than heroin! Addictive disease contributes to about 25 percent of all the deaths in the United States, and cigarette smoking is right up there beside cocaine, heroin, alcohol, and pill abuse as a leading cause of mortality.

Why tobacco is addictive is only partially understood.

One reason is that nicotine, an element of tobacco smoke, appears to be physically addictive. It's reinforcing psychoactive effects are thought to be what keeps smokers coming back for more. Smoking gets the nicotine quickly and effectively to the brain, its site of action. Nicotine seems to have its own "receptor sites" in the brain, which react to it when it enters the body. Opiates and Valium-like tranquilizers, called benzodiazepines, have similar, sensitive receptors in the brain that allow the drug to "work."

The reaction to nicotine is bodywide, causing the pulse rate to rise, blood pressure to elevate, brain waves to change, and hormones to be released, creating mood changes. Most smokers' brains interpret these to be positive or pleasurable. But too much smoking can also result in nausea and lightheadedness along with increased heart rate, which is actually an overdose of nicotine.

As a result of this receptor site binding action, smokers develop many of the same patterns of dependency that other drug addicts have. For example, smoking causes the body to develop a tolerance to cigarettes, requiring greater and greater "doses" (more cigarettes) just to achieve a "normal feeling."

Most cigarette smokers have to have a first smoke in the morning to get going. This is because that first cigarette, according to recent studies, sends a "burst" of nicotine to the brain that produces an initial feeling of mild pleasure. Most smokers then spend the rest of the day trying to duplicate that feeling by smoking more and more.

It's important also to remember that cigarette smoke contains a number of other elements that scientists also suspect may be addictive in the same way as nicotine. So no matter what "reduced ingredients" a cigarette ad promises, smoking itself is unhealthy. *Among other things, cigarette smoke contains cyanide, carbon monoxide, arsenous oxide, ammonia, and formaldehyde.*

Carbon monoxide is the same toxic stuff that's in your car's exhaust. The carbon monoxide from cigarettes tends to combine with the hemoglobin in the red blood cells. Hemoglobin carries the oxygen picked up in the lungs; when it is also carrying carbon monoxide, its capacity to carry oxygen is reduced by as much as 20 percent. That means the heart has to work harder to get the proper amount of oxygen to the body's tissue. The levels of carbon monoxide in a smoker are four to fifteen times higher than in a nonsmoker.

Cigarette smoke also produces "tars," which, when cooled in the lungs, form a brown sticky mess. While tars cause deterioration of your teeth, their direct link to lung cancer is a far more compelling reason to avoid cigarette smoke, both directly and indirectly.

Perhaps the worst part about cigarette addictiveness is that most scientists can only speculate about why it's so hard to stop. Only about 10 percent of all drinkers lose control of their alcohol habit to the point of repeated use in spite of the consequences. Recent surveys show that 75 percent of all smokers have tried to stop without success, despite all that is known about this "habit."

The physically addictive side of smoking is not the only reason why people can't stop. Smoking is very much a part of social activity in smokers' lives. Many people use cigarettes as props.

There is enormous peer group pressure among young people to smoke to be "one of the crowd." The young, who always feel immortal, also feel a natural curiosity about smoking. Cigarettes, although much more expensive than they used to be, are easily available to anyone of any age, despite laws that are supposed to limit sales to those over the age of 18 in most states.

People who use an addictive substance tend to use it either to help them through times of stress or when they have nothing else to do, when they are relaxing. Since the effects of cigarettes, unlike alcohol or drugs, are not immediately debilitating, smokers tend to light up at any time. What happens is that smokers unconsciously link smoking to common events—like deadlines which occur over and over in life, or even sitting around drinking coffee or watching TV. These events are called "triggers" and are discussed at greater length in Chapter Eight.

If you have had a heart attack or angina, the possible effect of cigarette smoking on your life is enormous. Each cigarette can cost you seventy-two minutes, so that every year you smoke can cost you eleven months. Every cigarette that you *don't* smoke increases your chances of living longer without getting another heart attack. If you're still smoking now, do some arithmetic and ask yourself if it's worth it.

There are other noncancerous but very serious problems caused by the action of cigarette smoke on the lungs and heart. The smoke damages hairlike structures in the respiratory tract called cilia. The cilia normally beat back and forth as fast as a thousand times a minute, moving mucus and other lubricants along the lining of the airways. The lubricants are important for normal respiratory functioning. One consequence of damaged cilia is bronchitis, a disorder characterized by a hacking cough in the morning upon waking up.

Depending on your age or sex, common respiratory ailments such as flu, colds, acute bronchitis, and pneumonia occur two to seven times more often in smokers than nonsmokers.

Another major lung disease related to cigarette smoking is emphysema, a condition in which pulmonary function is gradually but progressively diminished. Emphysema is an extremely debilitating disease; the afflicted person must struggle for every breath of air. Smokers have a greater chance of dying from this and other respiratory diseases.

WOMEN AND CIGARETTES

Cigarette smoking among women who also use oral contraceptives has been linked to a greater incidence of blood clot formation.

More women are smoking cigarettes than men these days, which is reflected in advertisements that pitch the "right" to smoke as a feminist issue. "You've come a long way, baby," is one recent example, although smoking has always been a sign of the liberated woman. This goes back to the days of the suffragist movement, when it was shocking to see a woman smoking a cigarette in a public place.

Given the proven risks to a woman's health, it's hard to see why these pitches work. In addition to the risks of heart and lung disease that women smokers face, there are special problems connected with pregnancy. The babies of women who smoke weigh less, and studies have shown that smoking during pregnancy increases the chances of birth defects and stillbirths. Other studies have shown that smoking might be connected with increased chances of spontaneous abortion. The message is clear and simple: Smoking and pregnancy don't mix.

Smoking and Pregnancy
Smoking during pregnancy can increase chances of smaller babies, birth defects, and stillbirths.

Health Risks of Smokers
1. Greater chances of heart disease
2. Much greater chances of lung cancer and long-term lung disease, such as bronchitis and emphysema
4. Greater chances of other cancers in the mouth, larynx, esophagus, kidney, bladder, and pancreas
4. Greater chances of ulcers
5. Greater chances of dying prematurely

Finally, there are some other risks that smokers ought to think about. If you smoke, your chances of dying before the age of 65 are twice as high as that of nonsmokers. You also have twice the risk of getting ulcers in your digestive tract. The list of health risks goes on and on. In fact, some experts calculate that *hundreds of thousands* of people die prematurely each year because they smoke.

RISKING THE HEALTH OF OTHERS

Another fact is, when you smoke you may also jeopardize the health of those around you, whether they smoke or not. In a poorly ventilated room, a nonsmoker can get a good dose of cigarette smoke. This kind of involuntary, or "passive," smoking might potentially be harmful to others who have heart problems, since a diseased heart is especially in need of oxygen.

Children are especially vulnerable to cigarette smoke. Infants of smoking parents have much greater chances of getting bronchitis or pneumonia. It's also more common for infants and young children of smoking parents to wheeze.

Young people are harmed by the example set by smoking parents:

Passive Smoking	
Cigarette smoking forces others to inhale harmful smoke whether they like it or not.	
Infants of smoking parents have much greater risks of lung disease.	Children of smoking parents are more likely to smoke than children of nonsmoking parents.

Children of smoking parents are much more likely to smoke than those of nonsmoking parents. Studies have been done on *10-year-olds who regularly smoke.* So, if you have children, do them a favor and kick the habit.

SMOKING IN THE WORKPLACE

Employers are beginning to recognize that nonsmoking employees are more productive than those who smoke. One study shows that smoking costs employers an average of $5,662 per year. This is because smokers tend to be absent more, have higher medical insurance costs, die younger, have decreased productivity from time spent smoking, and damage furniture and sensitive equipment.

Employers are also concerned because of the link between smoking and on-the-job accidents and the risk to nonsmoking employees from passive smoking.

New studies also demonstrate that certain occupations that expose workers to dangerous substances become more risky for those who smoke. For example, bus drivers, electricians, boilermakers, painters, roofers, firemen, asbestos and insulation workers, auto mechanics, plumbers, brick masons, taxidrivers, and printing press employees are all at greater risk for lung cancer than fellow employees who don't smoke. Their cancer risk is greater because smoking reduces their ability to clear industrial dust and other wastes from their lungs.

DRUGS AND SMOKING

Besides the effects of cigarettes on women who take the Pill, smoking also has a negative effect when combined with certain medications. While this information is not widely publicized, it is significant, especially for workers who must take certain medications. The drug-smoke interaction can be a result of certain elements of cigarette smoke, although no one is absolutely sure.

Some of the drugs whose effects are diminished by cigarette smoking include insulin (for diabetics), phenylbutazone (a painkiller used by arthritics), Inderal (a widely used heart drug), and theophylline (an antiasthmatic).

While the number of employers who insist on a smoke-free workplace is still minuscule, the movement is spreading. Tobacco is still the largest risk factor for cancer, and employers may find themselves the target of lawsuits from nonsmoking employees in the future. Already suits are being filed by a Washington, D.C., organization called Action for Smoking and Health. A smoke-free workplace may be a thing of the future, but that future may not be as far off as most people think.

CIGARETTES AND YOUR WALLET

Most people don't think about the costs of smoking when they light up. Perhaps they ought to, because the numbers are mind-boggling. First, there are the "big" costs from diseases caused by or related to cigarette smoking: hospitalization and medical care, days lost from work, and productivity loss due to premature death. These costs, which total in the *billions of dollars,* might be hard to imagine right now. So consider the expenses that come right out of your paycheck: the actual cost of a pack of cigarettes. Let's do some quick multiplication (we'll use $1.25 as the price of a pack of cigarettes):

If you smoke 1 pack per day, the yearly cost of your smoking habit is:	$ 456.25
If you smoke for 5 years, the cost would be	$2,281.25
If you smoke for 10 years, the cost would be	$4,562.50
If you smoke for 20 years, the cost would be	$9,125.00

If you took your cigarette money and put it in a piggybank, you'd have a lot of cash to play with—what would you do with it? Let's do the figuring again, this time for *two* packs of cigarettes a day:

If you smoke 2 packs per day, the yearly cost of your smoking habit is:	$ 912.50
If you smoke for 5 years, the cost would be	$ 4,562.50
If you smoke for 10 years, the cost would be	$ 9,125.00
If you smoke for 20 years, the cost would be	$18,250.00

Again, think about what you could do with that kind of money if it had been sitting in a Money Market account collecting hundreds of dollars' worth of interest. Isn't it a waste to see it go up in smoke?

Smoking Odors
Smoking leaves offensive odors in your home and car. It also dulls your taste buds.

GO SMOKELESS AND ODORLESS

Once you've been smoking for a while, your nose gets used to cigarette odors, so you don't notice the odor in your clothes and furniture. But nonsmokers do. In fact, many people who quit smoking are amazed at how noticeable and foul the smells of fresh smoke and stale cigarette butts can be. There's also the matter of your taste buds; when you quit smoking, you'll find that your sense of taste will be much keener. And that will mean that you'll get more enjoyment out of good food.

STRATEGY

KICKING THE HABIT—FOR GOOD

Many smokers want to quit but don't quite know how, are afraid of gaining weight, have tried and failed, or have succeeded for a short time and then started up again. Armed with some knowledge about what happens when you smoke and what happens when you quit will help you prepare for what you'll have to go through.

We think that nicotine is the main chemical in tobacco that stimulates your nervous system. Since it is also an addictive drug, once your brain is hooked on the stuff it requires a nicotine fix every twenty to thirty minutes. When you're having a "nicotine fit," the unpleasant feelings are caused by your system craving a substance that it has gotten used to. When you quit, your body has to readjust to a normal state in which it does not need nicotine. This is called withdrawal. It takes about a week for the body to readjust. During that time you might feel edgy, nervous, tired, nauseous, drowsy, irritable, disoriented, unable to sleep, or constipated. That is perfectly normal—you just have to ride it out.

Quitting Cigarettes and Not Gaining Weight

1. Stick to a healthy diet.
2. Snack on fruits and vegetables—have your snacks handy.
3. Chew sugarless gum or calorie-free mints if you need to put something in your mouth.

THE PSYCHOLOGICAL HURDLES

If it takes only a week to get over the nicotine addiction, why does it seem to take so much longer to really get over cigarettes? The answer is that the physical addiction to nicotine is just part of the picture. There are other things about cigarettes that are psychologically habit forming, like handling a cigarette and watching the smoke, using cigarettes as a crutch in uncomfortable situations, and feeling as if cigarettes give you an energy boost. Once you've actually gotten over the physical craving, it just takes time to get used to doing various activities without a cigarette in hand.

SMOKING AND WEIGHT GAIN

It's normal to gain between 5 and 10 pounds after quitting because eating seems to help the cigarette cravings. It seems that your metabolic rate tends to slow down when you quit because the stimulant effect of nicotine is absent.

There are a few things that you can do to keep from gaining weight without depriving yourself of satisfying your increased hunger (your hunger will get back to normal after a week or so). Follow the diet we've described in Chapter Six. Use vegetables and fruits as your snacks. Carry your vegetables around with you so that they're always handy. Also, some people find that chewing calorie-free mints or sugarless gum helps fill their need to have something in their mouth.

STRATEGY

MORE WAYS TO KICK THE HABIT

Surprisingly, 80 percent of the people who quit cigarettes do so by themselves without help from a program. But there are some very good programs that I would recommend if you want to spend up to $250 for help. At the end of this chapter is a list of recommended commercial stop-smoking programs. Quitting "cold turkey" is probably the best way, despite some period of nicotine withdrawal symptoms. Recently, a new antismoking gum, Nicorette, marketed by Merrell Dow Pharmaceuticals, has come on the market; it can help avoid those symptoms. You can obtain this gum only through prescription, and it should only be used on the instructions of your doctor. Nicorette is useful only after you've decided to quit and have done so. You must actually quit smoking altogether to benefit from this gum.

It's always a good idea to discuss any change in health behavior, such as quitting smoking, with your doctor. Because your physician knows you, he or she may have additional insights.

STRATEGY

SELF-HELP FOR SMOKERS

• Decide you really want to quit. There is nothing that can replace your resolve. Don't let anyone talk you out of it. Be positive about it:

1. Make a list of reasons why you should stop. Keep it with you and repeat it before you go to sleep at night.
2. Develop this list from all the reasons we've talked about in the chapter. You don't want to be an addict. You don't want to hurt other members of your family. You will be saving money. Anything you think will motivate you to get through the initial period of nicotine withdrawal.
3. Ask yourself each time you light up: Am I having so much fun that I'm willing to die for it? *Feel guilty about smoking!*

• Get into shape to quit. One of the best strategies for quitting is to also get into physical condition. As you know, it's hard to smoke and work out—smoking cuts your wind. So, as you get into shape, smoking will be less important.

• Ask someone to join with you. This isn't exactly a support group, but breaking a bad habit, is always easier with some support.

• Figure out *when* you smoke. Most people smoke at certain times. For example:

1. When they want to look busy
2. When they want to waste time (or feel busy)
3. In social situations
4. When they're embarrassed or looking for some way to feel comfortable in a social situation
5. When they're angry or upset or stressed
6. When they eat or drink
7. When the phone rings

These are known as "trigger situations." They can also be specific feelings, times of the day, or places.

Trigger situations can be countered by creating alternative actions: Make a list of your triggers and then create an alternative list:

If your trigger is drinking alcohol, stop drinking.

If your trigger is watching TV, go out instead.

If your trigger is the end of a meal, get up from the table quickly or end the meal with a food which makes cigarettes taste bad (like tea or milk).

If you routinely light up on a work break, change from coffee to tea or milk.

If you smoke at your desk, don't bring cigarettes to work.

Drink coffee instead of alcohol, and avoid sugar, which can create a craving. When you need an oral fix, have a carrot or celery stick.

Develop the kind of strategies you need to turn those triggers off, for example:

• Clean your house. Get rid of cigarettes, ashtrays, matches. Don't throw out those butts—rather, keep them in plain sight in a glass jar so you can see how disgusting smoking is.

• Celebrate every anniversary—be it a week or a month from the date you stop smoking.

• Set up a calendar. Mark off each "red letter" day you don't smoke. Display it and keep it close at hand.

Beating Alcohol and Drug Abuse Odds

Do you find that you absolutely need a drink or two at lunch to help you through the rest of the day? Do you need to get high on grass before you can relax enough to go to sleep? Do you need cocaine to get through the next big office meeting? If you find yourself relying more and more upon drugs (even sleeping pills) to help you cope with the stress of everyday life, you may be heading for disaster.

Drugs have become part of the American way of life. Over 22 million Americans have tried cocaine. Some 10 percent of high school seniors claimed to be daily users of marijuana. An estimated 7 percent of the adult population seriously abuses alcohol. Americans 14 and older drink an average of three gallons of liquor yearly, or 591 twelve-ounce beers, 115 bottles of wine, or 35 fifths of 80-proof liquor. An alcoholic's life span is shortened (on the average) by ten to twelve years. The *Harvard Medical Health Letter* has labeled alcoholism "the most devastating socio-medical problem faced by human society short of war and malnutrition." Substance abuse is now the nation's *third leading cause of death*—after heart disease and cancer. If you have a drug problem, you are not alone. But you and only you can decide to *do* something about your problem.

We are not suggesting that the *occasional* drink or two will immediately result in your imminent demise. However, if the occasional beer or two is now a six-pack or two, you could have a problem that is taking years off your life. The first thing you must do is honestly evaluate whether or not you have a problem.

WHAT IS SUBSTANCE ABUSE?

Substance abuse means the nonmedical misuse of any material for "psychic effect," which causes dependency or addiction.

Substance abuse refers not only to the misuse of illegal drugs like marijuana, cocaine, or heroin, but also to the misuse of legal drugs like Valium, Percodan, alcohol, or nicotine. (Cigarette smoking is so common that it requires a separate section; see Chapter Nine for more information). In reality, all of these substances are "drugs." But since the term "drug abuse" is commonly applied only to marijuana, heroin, cocaine, or LSD, the umbrella term "substance abuse" has evolved.

DO YOU HAVE A PROBLEM WITH SUBSTANCE ABUSE?

There are many complex reasons why people abuse alcohol and/or drugs. Quite a few doctors feel that a major reason for substance abuse is some sort of depression. Many people, some not even aware that they are depressed, find themselves turning to drugs to help them relax, elevate their mood, or simply to help them through the day. These people are depressed, and rather than learning how to cope or seeking professional help, they turn to substance abuse as an easy answer to solving their problems.

In some cases, depression results from an inability to handle stress correctly. (For more information on stress and how to cope with it, see Chapter Eight.) A person who cannot handle stress may feel inadequate and worthless. These feelings, in turn, may result in depression and, ultimately, in substance abuse.

In order to evaluate whether or not you have a substance abuse problem, take a few minutes and honestly answer the Personal Drug-Use Inventory (see below). If you find yourself answering yes to more than a few questions, then you may have a problem that needs immediate attention.

Personal Drug-Use Inventory

This list of questions can help you decide whether you are addicted to drugs or have the potential for addiction. There are no "good" or "bad" answers to many of them—only honest answers. But if you find yourself silently answering yes to more than a few, it may be time to start thinking about ways to reduce your use of drugs.

ARE DRUGS AFFECTING YOU FINANCIALLY?

- Has spending money on drugs kept you from buying necessities, such as food or clothing, or from paying the rent or mortgage?
- Do you worry about how you'll pay for the drugs you use?
- Have you ever borrowed money to buy drugs?

ARE DRUGS AFFECTING YOUR WORK?

- Have you ever missed a day's work because of using drugs?
- Have you ever used drugs for "fun" or to "help get through the day" while at work?
- Do your coworkers use drugs and try to get you to join them?
- Have you been worried lately about losing your job because of your use of drugs?

DO DRUGS GET YOU INTO TROUBLE?

- Have you ever driven a car while you've been under the influence of cocaine and/or drugs and/or alcohol?
- Have you ever had an accident or been given a ticket while you were using cocaine and/or drugs and/or alcohol?
- Have you lost a friend or friends because of your use of drugs?
- Do you lie about your drug use, even to your close friends?
- Do you sometimes argue with people about the way you use drugs?

WHAT ARE YOUR REASONS FOR USING DRUGS?

- Do you think about drugs at least once a day? More often than that?

ARE DRUGS AFFECTING THE WAY YOU THINK?

- Have you sometimes thought about suicide since you've been using drugs?
- Do you sometimes accept a drug without even wondering about its purity when a friend offers it to you?
- Are you unable to remember what happened after you've used drugs?
- Do you have trouble concentrating when you've taken drugs?

Drug Abuse Risks by Class

DRUG	PRIMARY NATURE OF DEPENDENCY	DEPENDENCY POTENTIAL	ORGAN DAMAGE OR DEATH RISK
Stimulants	Psychological	High	Moderate
Barbiturates	Physical	Moderate–High	Moderate–High
Benzodiazepines	Physical	Low	Low
Narcotic analgesics	Physical	High	Low
Alcohol	Physical	Moderate	High
Marijuana	Psychological	Low–Moderate	Low
Cigarettes	Physical–Psychological	High	High

Source: *The Little Black Pill Book,* ed. Lawrence D. Chilnick (New York: Bantam Books, 1983).

HOW COMMONLY ABUSED DRUGS AFFECT THE BODY

Generally, drugs are classified in groups by their principal action or effect on the central nervous system. Drugs that speed you up, like cocaine, amphetamines, caffeine, or nicotine, are called stimulants.

Drugs that calm you down, like benzodiazepines (Valium, etcetera) or barbiturates (Seconal, Tuinal, etcetera), are referred to as *sedative-hypnotics* or *depressants*. (Alcohol and other tranquilizers act as depressants.)

Drugs that relieve pain, like the opiates, opiate derivatives, or drugs such as morphine, Percodan, codeine, and Demerol are called *narcotic analgesics.*

All these substances work primarily by altering the brain's chemistry. When the drug reaches the brain, it affects the action of certain brain chemicals called neurotransmitters which are responsible for carrying nerve impulses across synapses (or connections) between cells. Essentially, these neurotransmitters act to speed up or slow down, to turn on or turn off the basic functions that influence our behavior.

When you use a drug, the neurotransmitters are switched on. Suddenly you're not quite as sleepy as you were before you inhaled the coke. In fact, the substance may actually replace the brain's own neurotransmitters. When this happens, the brain may "forget" to manufacture the neurotransmitter—after all, why should the brain do the work when the drugs you take do the same thing. This facet of the drug's biochemistry make it very difficult for a heavy user to stop taking some drugs. For example, the imbalance of neurotransmitters caused by heavy cocaine use may result in physical withdrawal symptoms when the user stops taking the drug: depression, paranoia, lethargy, insomnia, anxiety, and nausea and vomiting.

Many of these drugs have valid medical uses when administered under a physician's care. However, all of them have the potential for abuse which may result in addiction or dependency.

WHAT IS ADDICTION AND DEPENDENCY?

For decades, we all knew the classic definition of an addict. Addicts were "junkies," lying strewn in alleyways or deserted hallways, pitiful wrecks in complete agony willing to do anything for their next high. No respectable citizen would even know an addict, or at least would never admit to knowing one. Nowadays we know that addicts show up in the best of places. Like the Madison Avenue executive who was caught freebasing cocaine in her office. Or like the former First Lady, Betty Ford, who admitted she was addicted to prescription drugs. There have been numerous stories featuring the names of famous athletes and show biz personalities whose illnesses or even deaths have been connected to drug or alcohol abuse. Their prominence has significantly altered our ideas on this subject.

Addiction can no longer be relegated to our back alleys. Instead, we must confront it in every level of American society: the wealthy and the poor, the well-educated and the illiterate, legitimate business people and thieves.

Today we know that addiction is a disease. And, like other diseases, it can be treated.

The first sign of addiction is dependence.

This means a user begins to rely upon the drug to get through the week, to survive another day, to last one more hour. Without the drug, life is unbearable; with it, life can be enjoyed—that is dependence.

The next step toward addiction is increased tolerance to the drug.

This means the same amount of the drug you took before no longer has the desired effect. One or two "lines" of coke no longer gives you the same "rush" as before; now you need five, six, or more lines to get the same effect. You have developed a tolerance.

Addiction often follows dependence and increased tolerance.

For decades, addiction has been considered to mean that the body has a reaction when the drug is withdrawn. Severe headaches, nausea, vomiting, excessive mucus, or tremors in the absence of a drug would mean you were addicted. A strong desire for the drug would not be considered addiction.

Recently, the definition has broadened considerably to mean repeated and compulsive use of any substance despite adverse consequences. While addiction—in its new, more relevant definition—features dependency and tolerance, the key factor is "repeated use" despite adverse consequences.

Surprisingly, it is now known that some people can become dependent and even addicted to a drug when using very low doses, often no more than what a doctor may prescribe to treat an ailment. These people are among the 10 percent of the population who may have a genetic predisposition to addiction.

Some people are prone toward alcoholism, while others may be susceptible to tranquilizers or cocaine. At the moment there is no absolute way to tell who is genetically predisposed to addiction and dependency. But statistically, the knowledge of alcoholism's family pattern provides a clue to addiction chances with other drugs.

Dr. David Smith, of the Haight-Ashbury Free Clinic in San Francisco, reports that when one parent is an alcoholic, the chances of a son or daughter facing alcohol addiction are thirty-five times greater than for the general population. If both parents are alcoholics, the likelihood of alcoholism among their children increases by a factor of four hundred.

In fact, if you have a family or personal history of drug abuse of any kind, you are at greater risk of addiction than most people.

Even if you are not addicted or dependent, you run a greater health risk if you are even a "moderate" substance abuser.

OTHER RISKS ASSOCIATED WITH SUBSTANCE ABUSE

About Alcohol

- 50 percent of all deaths in automobile accidents are related to alcohol abuse.

- 50 percent of all homicides involve alcohol abuse.
- 25 percent of all suicides are related to alcohol abuse.
- The death rate for alcoholics from fire is ten times greater than for nonalcoholics.
- The suicide rate for alcoholics is six to fifteen times greater than that of the overall population.
- Alcohol causes chronic brain damage and is a source of mental deterioration in adults, second only to Alzheimer's disease.
- Cancer of the esophagus occurs at a rate up to seventeen times greater in alcoholics than among nondrinkers, while cancers of the mouth, tongue, and pharynx are also more common in alcoholics.
- Lower infant birth weights, IQs, and motor development are linked to drinking by pregnant women.
- Pedestrians with high blood levels of alcohol are twice as likely to be struck by a vehicle.
- Cirrhosis, the very serious and potentially fatal disease of the liver, will develop in 15 percent of all heavy drinkers.
- Large amounts of alcohol can cause alcoholic cardiomyopathy, a disease that damages the heart muscles.
- Alcoholics have a much higher incidence of peptic ulcers and pancreatitis than do nonalcoholics.
- The risk of dying from pneumonia is markedly increased in heavy drinkers.

OTHER DRUGS

Statistics listing the harmful effects of alcohol are so prevalent today largely because alcohol has been with us for so many years. (Nearly two hundred years ago, Benjamin Rush, M.D., called alcohol abuse a disease.) The people using cocaine, marijuana, and other potent drugs today are really acting as human guinea pigs for future generations, since the long-term side effects of these drugs may not be known for years to come. Unfortunately, for many it may be too late.

Many cocaine users are aware of the so-called minor health problems associated with snorting cocaine: a chronic runny nose, burns, inflammation, and even septal necrosis (the death of tissue separating the nostrils, causing a hole in the tissue and requiring surgical repair

—i.e., the "Teflon nose job"). But not everyone is aware that cocaine also increases the heart rate, raises blood pressure, speeds respiration, and raises blood sugar levels, conditions that can become very serious, even *fatal*.

Like cocaine, marijuana causes the heart to beat faster and work harder—a potentially dangerous effect for people suffering from hypertension or heart disease. Long-term marijuana use may also lead to bronchitis and lung cancer. Even if the risk of marijuana causing cancer is high, it will take many more years of study to establish a firm connection.

STRATEGY

BEATING SUBSTANCE ABUSE

Self-Help

If, after *honestly* and *realistically assessing your situation,* you conclude that you do not have a substance abuse problem, you may still wish to control your drinking or drug use. If this is the case, the following guidelines should help you prevent your substance abuse from getting out of control:

- Recognize and avoid situations where alcohol and/or drugs become the main focus of an activity, rather than an adjunct to it.
- Avoid drinking alcohol if you are taking other drugs.
- Set limits to your consumption of alcohol and drugs to protect your dignity and self-respect.
- Respect the person who chooses to abstain or drink in moderation.
- Provide food containing proteins, such as dairy products, fish, and meat, if you serve alcohol.
- *Never* drive after consuming alcohol or drugs; don't allow your family or friends to drive after drinking either.
- If you see symptoms of alcoholism or drug addiction, seek help immediately.
- Always make yourself available as a "chauffeur" for your teenage children so they'll call you before riding with a teenage friend who has been drinking!

Remember that one of the best ways to assure that you will not develop a substance abuse problem is to handle stress. Being able to cope successfully with stress will eliminate many of the reasons why people turn to alcohol or drug abuse in the first place. Please consult the strategies for dealing with stress in Chapter Eight.

But If You Do Have a Problem . . .

If you have a problem with substance abuse and you want to stop by yourself, remember that the safest way to get off any drug is to taper off slowly. The body and mind must have time to resume natural functioning once the drug has passed through the system.

Easing off drugs does take control, however, and with the more reinforcing drugs, like amphetamines or cocaine, it takes a strong will to make do with less each time. With these drugs it may be better to stop completely and avoid further exposure. But with drugs that cause physical dependency, like sedatives and benzodiazepines (i.e., Valium), stopping abruptly may not be safe.

Therefore, always consult your doctor or a detoxification program before stopping a prescription drug.

Professional Help

If you are unsure of how to go about getting off drugs, contact a doctor or enroll in a local drug treatment clinic or chemical dependency program. To find nearby programs, contact your state agency (see below) for more information. If you are seeing a psychotherapist to get off drugs, it is best to see a therapist referred to you by a local drug treatment clinic or organization; that way you'll ensure that your psychotherapist will be knowledgeable and sympathetic to your problem. Always make sure any psychotherapist you see for depression or substance abuse sends you to a competent physician for a complete physical exam. This is the only way you will ever know if your depression is being caused by some sort of underlying, serious physical condition whose symptoms are similar to depression!

Your company may provide an Employee Assistance Program (EAP) to help employees combat drug problems without fear of losing their jobs. Many companies and insurance policies have realized that it is far more cost-effective to stop alcohol- and drug-related problems in their earliest stages than to deal with the advanced stages of substance abuse. It is believed that this approach will improve production while combating the costs of ever-soaring insurance premiums, and the very real cost of having to replace a trained and experienced worker.

You should approach your shop steward, your company medical officer or nurse, or even have your own doctor contact the company to ensure that your rights are protected when you enroll in some sort of EAP.

Sources of Information on Drug Abuse Treatment Programs: State Agencies

ALABAMA
Division of Alcoholism and Drug
  Abuse
Department of Mental Health
135 South Union Street
Montgomery 36130
(205) 265-2301

ALASKA
Office of Alcoholism and Drug Abuse
Pouch H-05-F
Juneau 99811
(907) 586-6201

ARIZONA
Drug Abuse Section
Department of Health Services
2500 East Van Buren
Phoenix 85008
(602) 255-1239

ARKANSAS
Office on Alcohol and Drug Abuse
  Prevention
Suite 310
1515 West 7th Street
Little Rock 72202
(501) 371-2604

CALIFORNIA
Department of Alcohol and Drug
  Abuse
111 Capital Mall
Sacramento 95814
(916) 322-2974

COLORADO
Alcoholism and Drug Abuse Division
Department of Health
4210 East 11th Avenue
Denver 80220
(303) 320-8333

CONNECTICUT
Alcohol and Drug Abuse Commission
999 Asylum Avenue
Hartford 06105
(203) 566-4145

DELAWARE
Bureau of Alcoholism and Drug Abuse
1901 North DuPont Highway
Newcastle 19720
(302) 421-6101

DISTRICT OF COLUMBIA
Department of Human Services
Office of Health Planning and
  Development
601 Indiana Avenue, N.W.
Washington, D.C. 20004
(202) 724-5641

FLORIDA
Drug Abuse Program
1317 Winewood Boulevard
Tallahassee 32301
(904) 488-0900

GEORGIA
Alcoholism and Drug Abuse Section
Division of Mental Health & Mental
  Retardation
878 Peachtree Street
Atlanta 30309
(404) 894-4204

HAWAII
Alcohol and Drug Abuse Branch
1270 Queen·Emma Street
Honolulu 96813
(808) 548-7655

IDAHO
Bureau of Substance Abuse
450 West State
Boise 83720
(208) 334-4368

ILLINOIS
Dangerous Drugs Commission
300 North State Street
Chicago 60610
(312) 822-9860

INDIANA
Division of Addiction Services
Department of Mental Health
429 N. Pennsylvania
Indianapolis 46204
(317) 232-7816

IOWA
Department of Substance Abuse
505 Fifth Avenue
Des Moines 50319
(515) 281-3641

KANSAS
Department of Social Rehabilitation
  Services
Alcohol & Drug Abuse Services
2700 West Sixth Street
Topeka 66606
(913) 296-3925

KENTUCKY
Cabinet for Human Resources
Department of Substance Abuse
275 East Main Street
Frankfort 40621
(502) 564-2880

LOUISIANA
Office of Mental Health and Substance
  Abuse
P.O. Box 4049 ·
Baton Rouge 70821
(504) 342-2575

MAINE
Office of Alcoholism and Drug Abuse
  Prevention
32 Winthrop Street
Augusta 04330
(207) 289-2781

MARYLAND
State Drug Abuse Administration
201 West Preston Street
Baltimore 21201
(301) 282-7404

MASSACHUSETTS
Division of Drug Rehabilitation
160 North Washington Street
Boston 02114
(617) 727-8614

MICHIGAN
Office of Substance Abuse Services
Department of Public Health
3500 North Logan Street
Lansing 48909
(517) 373-8600

MINNESOTA
Chemical Dependency Program
    Division
Department of Public Welfare
568 Cedar
St. Paul 55155
(612) 296-4610

MISSISSIPPI
Division of Alcohol & Drug Abuse
Department of Mental Health
1102 Robert E. Lee State Office
    Building
Jackson 39201
(601) 359-1297

MISSOURI
Division of Alcoholism and Drug
    Abuse
Department of Mental Health
2002 Missouri Boulevard
P.O. Box 687
Jefferson City 65102
(314) 751-4942

MONTANA
Alcohol & Drug Abuse Division
Department of Institutions
1539 11th Avenue
Helena 59620
(406) 449-2827

NEBRASKA
Division on Alcoholism and Drug
    Abuse
P.O. Box 94728
Lincoln 68509
(402) 471-2851

NEVADA
Bureau of Alcohol & Drug Abuse
505 East King Street
Carson City 89710
(702) 885-4790

NEW HAMPSHIRE
State Alcohol & Drug Abuse Program
Hazen Drive
Concord 03301
(603) 271-4630

NEW JERSEY
Division of Narcotic & Drug Abuse
    Control
129 East Hanover Street
Trenton 08625
(609) 292-5760

NEW MEXICO
Substance Abuse Bureau
Behavioral Services Division
Crown Building
P.O. Box 968
Santa Fe 87503
(505) 984-0020

NEW YORK
Division of Substance Abuse Services
Executive Park South
Box 8200
Albany 12203
(518) 457-7629

NORTH CAROLINA
Alcohol and Drug Abuse Section
Department of Human Resources
325 North Salisbury Street
Raleigh 27611
(919) 733-4670

NORTH DAKOTA
Division of Alcoholism & Drug Abuse
Department of Human Services
State Capitol
Bismarck 58505
(701) 224-2767

OHIO
Bureau of Drug Abuse
65 South Front Street
Columbus 43215
(614) 466-9023

OKLAHOMA
Drug Abuse Services
Department of Mental Health
P.O. Box 53277, Capitol Station
Oklahoma City 73152
(405) 521-0044

OREGON
Department of Human Resources
Mental Health Division
Office of Programs for Alcohol & Drug
　Problems
2575 Bittern Street, N.E.
Salem 97310
(503) 378-2163

PENNSYLVANIA
Office of Drug and Alcohol Programs
Department of Health
Health and Welfare Building
Harrisburg 17108
(717) 787-9857

RHODE ISLAND
Division of Substance Abuse
Rhode Island Medical Center
Substance Administration Building
Cranston 02920
(401) 464-2091

SOUTH CAROLINA
Commission on Alcohol & Drug Abuse
3700 Forest Drive
Columbia 29204
(803) 758-2521

SOUTH DAKOTA
Division of Alcohol and Drug Abuse
523 East Capital
Joe Foss Building
Pierre 57501
(605) 773-3123

TENNESSEE
Alcohol & Drug Abuse Services
505 Deaderick Street
James K. Polk Building
Nashville 37219
(615) 741-1921

TEXAS
Drug Abuse Prevention Division
Department of Community Affairs
P.O. Box 13166
Austin 78711
(512) 443-4100

UTAH
Division of Alcoholism & Drugs
P.O. Box 2500
Salt Lake City 84110
(801) 533-6532

VERMONT
Alcohol & Drug Abuse Division
Department of Social & Rehabilitation
　Services
103 South Main Street
Waterbury 05676
(802) 241-2175

VIRGINIA
Division of Substance Abuse
Department of Mental Rehabilitation &
　Retardation
109 Governor Street
P.O. Box 1797
Richmond 23214
(804) 786-5313

WASHINGTON
Bureau of Alcohol & Substance Abuse
Department of Social & Health Services
　Office Building
Mail Stop OB-44W
Olympia 98504
(206) 753-3073

WEST VIRGINIA
Division of Alcohol and Drug Abuse
State Capitol
1800 Kanawha Boulevard East
Charleston 25305
(304) 348-3616

WISCONSIN
Office of Alcohol & Other Drug Abuse
P.O. Box 7851
One West Wilson Street
Madison 53707
(608) 266-2717

WYOMING
Division of Community Programs
Substance Abuse Programs
Hathaway Building
Cheyenne 82002
(307) 777-7118

PUERTO RICO
Department of Addiction Control
  Services
Alcohol and Drug Abuse Programs
Box B-Y, Rio Piedras Station
Rio Piedras 00928
(809) 763-5014

AMERICAN SAMOA
LBJ Tropical Medical Center
Department of Mental Health Clinic
Pago Pago 96799

GUAM
Mental Health & Substance Abuse
  Agency
P.O. Box 20999
Guam 96921

VIRGIN ISLANDS
Division of Mental Health, Alcoholism
  & Drug Dependency Services
P.O. Box 7329
St. Thomas 00801
(809) 774-7265

TRUST TERRITORIES
Director of Health Services
Office of the High Commissioner
Saipan 96950

Source: *National Directory of Drug Abuse and Alcoholism Treatment Programs.* (U.S. Department of Health and Human Services; National Institute on Drug Abuse and National Institute on Alcohol Abuse and Alcoholism)

Environmental Changes

Take the Personal Drug-Use Inventory (see page 140) and carefully evaluate your responses. You may notice that a definite pattern emerges. Most of your drug-taking might occur in work situations, for instance, or you may find that you consistently drive while under the influence of drugs. With this information, you will be able to focus on the aspects of your life that need the most attention.

Alcoholics Anonymous

Alcoholics Anonymous (AA), the grandfather of all self-help organizations, is run by recovering or recovered alcoholics. AA has a worldwide network and reaches into virtually every community in America. AA provides a specific program to follow as well the critical variable that most addicts require to get off and stay off drugs: each other. If you can find no local listing of AA, you can write to Alcoholics Anonymous, P.O. Box 459, Grand Central Station, New York, N.Y. 11017. In addition, there are related organizations, like Al-Anon, and Narcotics Anonymous and Pills Anonymous, which deal with other drugs besides alcohol.

Therapeutic Communities

Therapeutic communities are nonmedical self-help programs based originally on the Synanon model, the California therapeutic community founded in the late 1950s. Today, therapeutic communities vary widely, from cultish communities revolving around a charismatic leader to communities established to help medical professionals change their own drug habits. Because therapeutic communities are so different, it is essential to inspect them closely. Find out how they are run, who is on their board of directors, what their goals and values are, whether they have medically trained professionals on their staff, and their follow-up success rate.

Beating the Odds of Accidental Injury

Most people are surprised to learn that accidents cause more premature deaths among Americans each year than do illness. As for other types of premature death, risk factors for injuries can be identified and diminished, and in many cases eliminated altogether. If you spend time identifying the potential hazards of everyday life, you can, with some effort, beat the odds.

WHAT ARE THE RISKS?

Accidents, in general, are the number-one cause of death among young people under age 44. Each year, over 100,000 Americans are killed in accidents and 10 million are disabled. Auto accidents (including pedestrian accidents) are the overall leading cause of accidental death, accounting for over half of all fatalities, and about 20 percent of the injuries. Therefore, driving safety is one of the most important areas to consider as a risk factor. But auto accidents are by no means the only potential risk.

Nonfatal accidents in the home equal the number of auto and work-related injuries, though as a society we pay far more attention to auto and job safety. Ironically, we have much more control over accidents than we think.

Most people think that accidents "happen." This is a myth. If you recognize potential hazards, if you "live defensively" and modify your habits to protect yourself and your children, you can prevent most accidents from happening.

Just as a healthy diet and exercise should be a part of your everyday diet, safety should also be a part of the way you practice health.

WHY DO WE HAVE ACCIDENTS AND INJURIES?

There are many reasons why accidents that cause injury occur, and there are several leading risk factors, including age, sex, developmental abilities, emotional states, and drunkenness.

We know that older people and younger people have more accidents. The elderly suffer falls, pedestrian injuries, and burns more frequently due to impaired eyesight, weakness, loss of coordination, and drug interactions that may cause dizziness. The causes of accidents among the elderly are relatively straightforward compared to those of children.

For example, boys have more injuries than girls, and more infants die in auto accidents than older children. Adolescents are more frequent victims of suicide and homicide than elementary school children.

Are certain kids "accident-prone"? Experts say that a number of physical and psychological traits among "child accident repeaters" can be identified. Most are risk takers, impulsive, careless, or have certain coordination problems related to depth perception or reactive abilities. Other factors relate to developmental characteristics such as the intelligence, experience, and judgment of the child.

Studies have also discovered that children under certain types of personal and family stress are more likely to have accidents. It's possible they may have repeated exposure to hazards because of their parents' marital discord, parental preoccupation with their own problems, or a child's preoccupation with the parents' problems.

Children generally have more accidents because they are just learning to be social, to test their physical skills, and they are exposed to more "environmental" hazards: poisons, bike riding, hot food spilling, heavy objects on shelves or tables. Some haven't developed enough coordination for certain athletic activities they participate in during school or recreation, such as using gymnastic equipment or playing a team sport beyond their skill level.

Teens are often involved in accidents because they don't think of the consequences of choices they make and fall into peer pressure, which may lead to risk-taking behavior. Some are connected to auto use and others to amateur sports, and drug or alcohol use. Almost all involve the level of maturity or sense of judgment of the individuals.

Sex differences also figure in accidents, since males, statistically, are at higher risk for all types of accidents. Even though men are often more frequently exposed to dangerous situations, they don't have more on-the-job accidents. However, life-style differences between males and females in most sectors of society do contribute to a higher level of injuries for men. For example, men do more driving, more drinking, and engage in more dangerous sports, such as hunting, skydiving, boating, and so on, than women.

One other very important factor in susceptibility to injury is the use of alcohol. This has been well documented as a risk factor in recreational boating, motor vehicle crashes, swimming, falls, fires, and for pedestrians.

STRATEGY

PREVENTING ACCIDENTS

Most of us could be protected from accidents during common behavior that we repeat frequently. For example, do you remember to use your seat belt every time you get into your car? Do you remember to test the temperature of your tap water before you put your child in the tub?

The best strategies to prevent an injury are those that will protect us *regardless* of our behavior: using automatic seat belt restraint systems or air bags that automatically inflate on impact, or having your hot water heater turned down to a safe level so that you don't have to remember to test the water each time. It would be best if all hot water heaters were manufactured so that they would not heat above 130 degrees; then you would get rid of all tap water scaldings. But since it's unlikely that this requirement will happen soon, we have to take our own steps to protect ourselves.

In general, it's the *frequency* of actions that an individual must take to protect himself that makes it difficult to prevent injuries. Preventive strategies should focus on life-style and changes in the home environment that make us less subject to human factors of delay, discomfort, forgetfulness, and cost.

Generally, we may recognize situations that involve potential dangers and hazards but feel "it can't happen to me," or "it will never happen to me." So we take chances and procrastinate before making positive changes. We feel that it is better to be safe than sorry, but don't translate our words into action. The main objective of any injury prevention strategy should be to identify any existing hazard and then take action to break a certain chain of events that may lead to injury.

KEEPING YOUR KIDS SAFE

"Safety engineering" by parents will always be a primary means of preventing injuries to young children. This means being able to avoid injury by anticipating what your children's abilities to hurt themselves might be. The most important tip for keeping infants and toddlers safe is never to assume that a child's motor abilities will remain the same from day to day.

For example, if you have an infant crawling around on his or her hands and knees, check items that are at the child's eye level and then move the potentially dangerous ones. Don't just say: "I will be very careful about watching my child around this particular thing."

Supervision should not be the main form of protection against injury except in very young children. Supervision alone isn't the solution.

Often parents are absent-minded and careless. It is much easier to make the environmental change. Then it's done—you don't have to worry about constant monitoring of a young child.

• Use "stay away" toddler gates at the top and bottom of the stairs rather than constant supervision.
• Make sure there aren't sharp edges on children's toys.
• Buy only flame-retardant clothing.
• Buy only age-appropriate toys, and monitor their use. Infants and young toddlers should not play with small toy parts of an older sibling.
• Keep food in original containers—don't put potentially harmful food in candy jars, etcetera.
• Be certain that dangling cords from coffee makers, toasters, etcetera are out of reach. *Never* leave a child unattended in the kitchen.

Use extra care when heating foods for or around your child. Safe means keeping pot handles turned in, testing temperatures of food, especially microwaved food, and keeping your child in a safe place while cooking.

• Keep razors, scissors, and other sharp instruments in a closed, secure place. A medicine cabinet is not always out of a child's reach and should have a safety lock. Even shampoos and colognes can be harmful.

• Read warning labels and directions before using a product for the first time. Be aware that antidotes and labels are often outdated or incorrect on different kinds of toxic products.

• Everyone should have a basic first-aid kit in a box in the home, but it should be out of the reach of children. It should have emergency phone numbers such as the Poison Control Center's number pasted to the lid (emergency numbers should be posted beside a telephone as well). And it should contain syrup of ipecac, to administer in certain poisoning incidents when directed to do so by medical staff.

Commerical enterprise has led to a large number of safety items being marketed for the home; items specifically designed to protect young children within their environment. Every home should have some safety equipment just as a basic component.

• Smoke detectors, fire extinguishers, and a portable escape ladder for fires are a must.

• For young children you will want to explore a variety of products like stove or fireplace guards and cabinet locks, as well as more standard first-aid products like splints and braces.

• All states have infant or toddler automobile seat laws. Make sure that, at the very least, you comply with the law; go one step further and get the best possible equipment. This is not the place to try for a bargain (other than a discount price). Most states, through the State Health Department, have a child auto safety program and resource center, which will be helpful in picking out infant and toddler seats.

• Don't be tempted to forgo lead testing of your child by thinking of lead paint poisoning as an "inner city" problem. Families who purchase and renovate old houses have a particularly high rate of lead-poisoned children.

• Likewise, be careful about buying secondhand furniture for infants and young children. Make sure that it meets all post-1973 codes and standards, and that it is in good repair. For example, you really don't want to buy an antique highchair that is either rickety or does not have restraining straps to prevent the child from falling. Check with your state regional office of the Consumer Product Safety Commission.

• Don't put children's furniture or cribs near windows. Don't put them near other furniture which they can climb onto. Don't cover a mattress with a plastic bag that could cause suffocation.

• Make sure that the crib mattress fits snugly, with not more than a two-finger gap between mattress and crib.

• Remove dangling cords that might entangle children.

• Children should be taught basic safety behaviors. In fact, both children and the family should be trained within the scope of their age limitations to recognize dangers.

• Parents must set an example for basic safety behaviors that will carry children on into their later life through their teenage years.

• Setting other general examples for children—like wearing seat belts—that will be carried on later in life in an important safety measure, too. Since there is just no excuse not to wear a seat belt, parents should make it mandatory that the car doesn't move unless everyone is buckled up. This should be done even for short rides, because most car injuries and deaths occur close to home and at low speeds.

• Children should definitely be taught what to do in case of a fire, especially children under the age of 5, who might not know what to do and might hide if a fire occurred.

• There should be an escape plan in case of fire for all family members so that they know how to get out of each room. Practice the plan at night, which is when most fires occur. Children should be taught to crawl under smoke, not to go back for a pet, and to meet at one place should a fire break out. They should be told not to touch a door first but to see if it is hot; they must be taught the drop-and-roll technique for putting out flames on clothes.

Children really need to practice safety behavior; it's not effective just to tell them "don't do this or that." The focus should always be on positive behavior.

• Avoid saying "Don't play with matches" or "Don't touch matches." That may only arouse curiosity. Use a positive approach and tell the child, "Always give me any matches or lighters that you find." This gives the child a point of action to take when confronted with a dangerous situation. It also gives the adult the opportunity to praise the child and reinforce a positive behavior.

• Other safety behavior that should be taught includes:

1. How to swim. No child should be unable to swim. The earlier you start a child in the water, the better. Try, if at all possible, to get a child professional teaching at the YMCA or elsewhere. This is one of the most valuable safety measures any parent can take.

   If there is a pool on your property or in your neighborhood, make sure it is fenced and locked against entry by an unattended child. If you own a pool, purchase a floating alarm system.

2. The basic rule of the road for bikes is the same for automobiles; you need to ride defensively. Parents may need to set limits on the use of bikes so that they are not used on well-traveled roads until the child can follow rules of the road properly.

3. Begin teaching pedestrian safety early. Teach your children how to cross streets properly.

• Don't go out and buy the top-of-the-line bike for your child if it's not the right size. And don't turn children loose in the street with their bikes without first teaching them basic safety rules. If you can get a child to wear a bike helmet, that's the best measure, but there is a lot of peer pressure against it in this country.

• Besides injuries in the home, children can often be injured by toys, especially those with sharp points or ones that shoot projectiles that can harm an eye or be swallowed. If your child has a toy such as this and is injured, report it to the Consumer Product Safety office nearest you. You can look it up in the phone book under "Consumer Protection," or you can call the U.S. Consumer Product Safety Commission at 800-638-2772. Toy chests should have a safe closing mechanism or no lid at all.

• Kids are often injured in the playground—especially when unattended—and in school sports. Playground injuries tend to be a result of a foreign body like a rock or stick. More serious injuries occur from falls on hard playground surfaces. Check your playground for safety surfaces under swings, etcetera. School sports injuries often are a result of poor coaching, poor training, and poor attention to injuries. Before letting your child participate in a school sport, check it out. Talk to the coach, other parents. Make sure that your child has a complete physical exam before participating. Make sure that the coaches are qualified, not just a math teacher looking for a few extra dollars.

You can't expect your child to use appropriate safety behavior if you don't yourself.

• You can also set an example by wearing safety goggles for home workshop activities, where a lot of eye injuries happen to adolescents.

• Setting an example also relates to drugs and alcohol use, among teens especially. If you can set only one kind of example, don't drive while impaired from drugs or alcohol. Your child certainly won't pay any attention to your admonitions if you don't practice what you preach.

KEEPING YOURSELF SAFE

• Everyone should wear a seat belt. More than twenty states now have "buckle up" laws. This is the number-one way to prevent auto injuries. There are reams of data that demonstrate that seat belts save lives, especially in accidents under 35 miles per hour, which are the most frequent. In states where seat belts are mandatory, automobile fatalities have been cut by 30 percent. Information on seat belts and highway safety can be obtained from the National Highway Traffic Safety Administration, NTS-10 400 7th Street S.W., Washington, D.C. 20590, or your state governor's highway safety bureau.

Other highway and driving safety steps are:

• Don't ever drive and drink or drive and take drugs. Be especially careful if you are using a prescription pill that may make you drowsy or affect your reflexes. Always check with your doctor.

• Observing the 55-mile-per-hour speed limit also saves many thousands of lives each year.

• Motorcycle accidents account for five times more fatalities than autos—so if you're going to ride a cycle, always wear protective headgear. Accidents without helmets cause three to five times as many fatalities.

• Consider some adult safety engineering in the home. Use a safety checklist to identify things that need to be changed.

To prevent falls:

1. Keep heavy traffic areas well lit and clean of all obstacles such as furniture and toys.
2. Install night lights in bathrooms, bedrooms, hallways, and other areas family members might walk through during the night.
3. Have light switches at both top and bottom of stairs.
4. Do not use stairs to store anything—even for short periods of time.
5. Use nonskid mats in bathtubs, alongside toilets, etcetera.

6. Firmly affix every railing.
7. Loose throw rugs should be firmly secured and made skidproof.
8. Make sure extension cords are taped down or placed under rugs or between furniture and walls. Make sure you have no frayed cords.

A lot of accident prevention requires common sense, and there are many measures you can take that are simple:

You can prevent fires and burns:

1. When cooking, keep pot handles turned inward.
2. Don't leave hot liquids where kids can reach them—especially toddlers, who are always "exploring." Don't carry hot liquids and a child at the same time.
3. Use smoke detectors and install them properly in stairwells, in hallways and outside bedrooms, at the head of basement stairs, and at the foot of stairs to upper floors. Replace the battery on your birthday to remember. Studies have shown that fatalities can be avoided in over 90 percent of all fires if smoke detectors are working and present. *Also, don't smoke in bed and don't leave cigarettes lying around in ashtrays to burn out.*
4. Plan and practice escape routes in case of fire. Don't assume "it can't happen to me."
5. Keep escape ladders in rooms where necessary and remember to crawl under smoke. If your clothes catch fire, drop to the ground and roll. Use cold water for any type of burn.
6. Use shock stops or safety plugs in unused wall outlets.
7. Hair dryers, radios, etcetera, should not be left plugged in and should never be near water.
8. Keep a fire extinguisher in a handy place to put out a small fire or clear an escape path.
9. When using flammable liquids, make sure there is adequate ventilation and that they are away from any source of ignition, such as a pilot light or a cigarette.
10. Keep your basement a safe environment. All poisonous substances must be kept out of reach of kids if they share the basement for a playroom.
11. If you use a space heater, see that it is stable with a protective covering, at least 36 inches from curtains, paper, and furniture. It must be properly plugged into its own outlet.

• Keep all flammable liquids stored properly. Read the label and check with your salesman when you buy a dangerous substance. Make sure there is adequate ventilation in the basement.
• The same goes for laundry liquids and detergents, which are especially dangerous to children.

• If you keep tools in the basement, keep them stored properly.

• Obviously, this goes for firearms, too. Keep all guns in a locked cabinet.

Poisonings can also be prevented simply:

• Never underestimate a child's ability to get into any locked area or package. Keep all dangerous medicine and household cleaning supplies on high shelves even if they have child-resistant caps. Children can mistake bottles that look like food but are really poison.

• Don't refer to medicine as "candy" when trying to convince a child to take some. If the child believes you, he or she may not ask you when some medicine is lying around unattended.

• Keep plants out of the reach of children. Some plants can actually cause fatalities when nibbled. Learn the names and toxicity of your plants.

• If you suspect poisoning, call your doctor or Poison Control Center first. Many poisonings can be treated first over the phone.

• Keep ipecac syrup in the house to induce vomiting, but use it only when instructed by a doctor or Poison Control Center.

• Know what to do in the event an injury does occur. Have a first-aid kit and book on hand for adult injuries. Learn CPR and other emergency measures, like the Heimlich maneuver. Call your doctor first if you can; procedures recommended in the books are sometimes outdated. It may also be better to call a Poison Control Center first rather than to follow the book's suggestion. (This number is listed in your phone book. Obtain it and post it near your phone.)

• Think of yourself as a consumer advocate for products you bring into your home. When you identify a hazardous product, get in touch with the agency that can do something about recalling or changing the design of that product such as the U.S. Consumer Product Safety Commission (800-638-2772).

• Do a systematic room-by-room check of the house, the garage, the basement, and other property for safety hazards. Examine the accessibility of potentially dangerous items to make necessary changes.

Avoiding Recreational Injuries

• Make sure all your sports equipment is in good working order.

• As with children, adults should know the rules of the road for bicycling. These rules should be observed and obeyed.

Household Safety Inventory

CHECK YOUR HOUSE:

OUTSIDE
Porches and balconies in good repair?
Stairs in good repair?
Hand railings in good repair?

KITCHEN
All appliances properly installed?
Household cleaning products out of reach of children?
Emergency phone numbers posted near telephone?
Matches, lighters out of reach of children?
Appliance cords out of reach of children?
Knives and other dangerous appliances out of reach?
Snacks not stored on or above stove?
Shock stops on unused electrical outlets?

STAIRS
Toddler gates at top and bottom of stairs?
Railings and stairs in good repair?

BATHROOM
Water set lower than 125° F?
Medicine cabinet locked or inaccessible to children?
Medicine in proper, childproof containers?
Medicine properly labeled?
Electrical appliances stored away from washbasin, tub, and shower?
No electrical space heater?
Shock stops in empty outlets?
Razors, shaving equipment out of reach of children?
Toxic shampoos, soaps, cosmetics out of reach of children?

BEDROOMS
CHILDREN'S ROOMS:
  Shock stops on all unused outlets?
  Crib in good repair?
  Slats on cribs spaced at intervals less than 2⅜"?
  Strings, cords, games out of reach from crib?
  Bumper guards on crib?
  Mattress fits crib properly?
  No plastic bags on pillows, mattress, etcetera?
  Window guards, locks, bars properly installed?
  Cribs, bed away from windows?

Household Safety Inventory (cont.)

ADULT ROOMS:

Shock stops on all electrical outlets?

Extension cords inaccessible to children?

Matches, lighters out of reach of children?

Cosmetics out of reach?

No dangling cords or extension cords?

BASEMENT

Poisonous substances stored out of reach?

Tools, power cords put away?

Flammable liquids properly labeled and stored?

Proper wiring installed?

All boilers, oil tanks, et cetera, properly operating?

Stairs in good repair?

Railings and walls in good repair?

All fuses or electrical grounds properly installed?

GENERAL

Smoke detectors properly installed with fresh batteries?

Working fire extinguishers?

Potentially toxic plants out of reach of children?

Nonlead paints used on walls?

First-aid kits and ipecac syrup on hand?

Halls and stairways properly lit?

All wiring meets regulations?

Electrical sockets not overloaded?

Extension cords properly secured?

No dangling cords?

Protection around woodstove or fireplace?

Cigarettes, lighters, ashtrays out of reach of children?

Source: Massachusetts State Childhood Injury Prevention Program.

1. If you ride at night, wear white and have reflective materials attached to the bike.
2. If a young child is going to ride on your bike, use a properly installed seat and belt to prevent falls and to keep limbs from getting caught in the spokes. Infants under six months should not go on bikes.
3. Whether you bike, roller-skate, or jog, don't wear headphones which prevent you from hearing cars or other hazards.
4. Ride with the traffic on the right side of the road.

• Water safety is another area where adults should be as careful as children. Know water safety measures.

1. Never dive headfirst into unfamiliar waters or a shallow pool.
2. Never swim alone or after drinking alcohol, or in a restricted area.
3. When boating, make sure there is a life jacket or flotation device for every person in the boat.

• You can prevent amateur sports injuries by consulting your doctor whenever you begin a new sport. Before you begin any sort of exercise, make sure you have warmed up properly by stretching. Cool down gradually after any exercise.

STRATEGY

FIND A GOOD CONSUMER ORGANIZATION

There are a number of organizations or consumer groups which help protect you from harm. The U.S. Consumer Product Safety Commission (800-638-2772) is a good place to get information, but also it is a place where people can complain about hazardous products.

Almost every state has a Poison Control system and most of these have an emergency hotline. The number should be posted near your phone and kept in the first-aid kit.

There are many support groups for those already seriously injured, like the National Society for Head Injury in Washington, D.C., and the American Foundation for the Blind, 15 West 16th Street, New York, N.Y. 10011, (212) 620-2000.

Others to contact:
• National Highway Traffic Safety Administration (800-424-9393).
• Local Red Cross chapters.
• American Academy of Pediatrics (800-336-5475).

Of course, the most effective strategy is legislation that requires certain preventive behaviors and actions. But whether this will happen or not remains to be seen. Childproof closures on medications and on some household products, under the Poisoning Prevention Act, were effective as were other laws that limited the number of aspirin in a children's bottle. Those laws were both effective in reducing the number of deaths from poisonings to young children. Other examples of needed legislation that has finally been enacted are rules for flame-retardant sleepwear and banning fireworks in many states. In high schools, mandatory facial protection for hockey goalies has resulted in their having far fewer facial injuries than other hockey players.

But remember, once again, strategies for beating the odds of injury and accident begin with your own common sense and your ability to perceive a potentially dangerous situation, and then your desire to make positive environmental changes in your home that will keep you and your family safe.

General Diet Tips to Beat the Odds

Within the last few years, Americans have been deluged with advice —sometimes conflicting—on what they should or should not eat. Practically every day we're told to eat more fiber, less salt, more polyunsaturated fats, less polyunsaturated fats, more calcium, less cholesterol, more vegetables, less red meat. . . . The list of what we should or should not eat is endless—even if you're one of the lucky ones who do not have to lose weight. What should you do if you want to have a healthy diet without necessarily losing weight?

This chapter examines this question along with some of the more popular "hot topic" diet strategies—like eating more fiber—within the context of an overall healthy, nutritious diet. Remember, you don't have to be overweight to eat a good diet. The quality of the food you eat is important, since it may ultimately result in a longer, healthy life for you.

HOT TOPIC #1: FIBER

Fiber has been with us for longer than we might think. You may remember your parents urging you to eat your roughage (such as lettuce), since it was good for your "system" (i.e., bowels). What our parents used to call "roughage" is now called "fiber." Eating more roughage was—and still is—an effective way to combat constipation. However, many doctors now believe that fiber may be an important tool against many other conditions, ranging from heart disease to cancer.

What Is Fiber?

Fiber is the indigestible material found in plants, primarily in the cell walls, that give a firm structure to the plant. Meat, no matter how tough, is not a source of fiber. Fiber cannot be digested; it passes almost completely intact from the mouth to the large intestine. In the large intestine, some forms of fiber may be fermented by bacteria, which may result in a temporary condition of intestinal gas. Fiber may absorb water, much like a sponge, resulting in larger, softer stools that pass easily and quickly through the rectum. (This is how fiber earned its reputation as nature's laxative.) Fiber occurs in many forms: bran and many fruits, beans, vegetables, and cereals are all considered good sources of fiber.

The typical American consumes about 15 grams of fiber a day. Many doctors believe that we would be healthier eating 35 to 40 grams a day. While I believe in the importance of fiber, I personally do not set fiber-consumption goals for my patients. Rather, I encourage them to eat more fiber as an important part of a healthy and nutritious diet. But refrain from going fiber-crazy; too much fiber can prevent the body from absorbing important minerals. Any increase in fiber should be done gradually, not overnight. It is important to consult your doctor before embarking on any major diet change, especially since a high-fiber diet is not for everyone. The elderly, people who suffer from bowel disorders, kidney disease, diabetes, or those who are undernourished may encounter serious problems on a high-fiber diet.

Fiber-Rich Foods

Whole grains, fruits, and vegetables form the most common sources of fiber in our diets. In addition, commonly used food additives, such as pectins and gums, normally added to improve texture and thickness in processed foods, are also considered fiber. A fiber-rich diet doesn't mean that you are forced to eat "tree-bark" for the rest of your life.

You may be surprised to find out that apples, grapefruits, pears, strawberries, cucumbers, and peas all contain healthy amounts of fiber (see box on page 171 for foods rich in fiber). A fiber-rich diet is quite appetizing.

Benefits from Fiber

As stated earlier, the importance of fiber as a laxative has been known for many years. By absorbing water in the bowels, fiber promotes the smooth, efficient passage of feces through the intestines. A high-fiber diet also results in quicker elimination of food—people on a high-fiber diet pass food through their system in an average of 36 hours, while those on a low-fiber diet take an average of 77 hours.

Intestinal Disorders

The ability to pass feces smoothly and without much effort is believed to lessen the chance of developing disorders of the colon and rectum, such as *hemorrhoids* and *diverticulosis* (formation of pockets in the large intestine that may become infected and inflamed).

Diabetes

A high-fiber, high-complex-carbohydrate diet may also be helpful in controlling *diabetes*. In fact, in one study, diabetics following this diet were able to lessen their need for insulin to the level where some diabetics were able to stop taking insulin. It appears that fiber hinders the absorption of carbohydrates, thereby preventing high blood sugar levels from occurring.

Weight Loss

A high-fiber diet may also help you lose weight. Fiber fights obesity because:

- Fiber contains few calories, and fiber-rich foods usually are low in calories.
- Since fiber absorbs water, you are more likely to feel "full" after consuming a high-fiber food.
- Most fiber-rich foods take longer to eat, lessening the chance of your overeating.

- Since fiber "pushes" food through your system, small amounts of fat and protein are excreted rather than absorbed.
- Fiber is usually very bulky and makes you feel full without consuming a tremendous amount of calories.

Fiber and Cholesterol

Some forms of fiber may actually lower cholesterol levels, thereby reducing your risk of heart disease. The type of fiber you eat is very important. Bran, which is almost all cellulose (a type of fiber), has no positive effect on your cholesterol level (bran may actually raise your cholesterol). However, a significant lowering of cholesterol may be achieved by eating other fiber-rich foods, such as fruits (containing pectins), beans (which contain guar gum), rolled oats, and carrots. One study reported that eating 7 ounces of raw carrots for breakfast over a three-week period could result in an 11 percent reduction in cholesterol levels. (For more information on reducing cholesterol, see Chapter Six.)

STRATEGY

EATING MORE FIBER

If you want to increase your fiber consumption, make sure you eat a wide variety of fibrous foods in the proper amount. (Please consult the following box for a list of fiber-rich foods.)

A high-fiber diet should be a part of an already healthy, nutritious diet. Sprinkling bran over a pint of ice cream won't do you much good.

Add fiber to your diet gradually; don't O.D. on bran the first day. A reasonable increase in fiber will allow your body to adjust properly to the higher fiber levels. How much fiber should you eat? That depends on many factors, such as your age, overall health, and weight —ask your doctor to recommend an amount for *you*.

To prevent constipation, drink plenty of liquids when eating fiber.

When buying breads and cereals, look for the words "whole grain," "whole wheat," or "whole oats" on the label or ingredients list.

Raw fruits and vegetables are more fiber-rich than steamed, peeled, cooked, or otherwise altered fruits and vegetables. Try to eat a salad each day.

Some Examples of Foods with High Fiber Content

FOOD	SERVING SIZE	FIBER (GRAMS)
All-Bran Cereal	1 cup	23.0
Bran Buds	¾ cup	18.0
Grape Nuts	⅓ cup	5.0
Shredded Wheat	2 biscuits	6.1
Apple	1 small	3.1
Banana	1 medium	1.8
Grapefruit	½	2.6
Grapes	16 raw	.4
Pear	1 med. raw	2.8
Strawberries	½ cup	2.6
Tangerine	1 medium	2.1
Beets	⅔ cup cooked	2.1
Cabbage	¾ cup cooked	2.2
Cabbage	1 cup raw	2.1
Carrots	1 medium	3.7
Celery	2½ stalks raw	3.0
Corn kernels	⅔ cup	4.2
Green peppers	1 large raw	2.4
Kidney beans	1 cup cooked	3.6
Lentils	½ cup cooked	4.0
Parsnips	¾ cup cooked	5.9
Peas	½ cup cooked	3.8
Zucchini	½ cup cooked	2.5

Source: *Jane Brody's Nutrition Book* (New York: Bantam Books, 1982).

Remember, it is important to consult with your doctor before undergoing any major diet change. For the majority of people, a high-fiber diet poses no problems; however, there are some people—especially those who suffer from bowel disorders, kidney disease, or diabetes, or those who are undernourished—for whom a high-fiber diet may not be advisable. Please ask your doctor whether he or she recommends a high-fiber diet for you before you embark on one.

HOT TOPIC #2: FAT

Recently, more and more people have become aware of the need to reduce fat intake in their diet. And yet Americans still consume 30 percent more fat today than they did in 1910—42 percent of the typical American diet consists of fat. I, along with the National Academy of Sciences and the American Heart Association, recommend that fat consumption be lowered to 30 percent. Others, such as the late Nathan Pritikin and the Center for Science in the Public Interest, recommend fat consumption be reduced to 10 percent of your daily calorie intake.

An even more important change concerns the *type* of fat you consume. Dietary fat largely consists of three types of fatty acids, called saturated, monosaturated, and polyunsaturated. Many animal fats contain mainly saturated fats, while vegetable fats contain a high amount of monosaturated and polyunsaturated fats.

Saturated fats increase the amount of "bad" cholesterol in your blood, while polyunsaturated fats lower these "bad" cholesterol levels. In general, most blood fat problems (e.g., high cholesterol and triglyceride levels) will require restriction of calories first, *then* a change in the type of fats you consume.

"Good" and "Bad" Cholesterol

Cholesterol can be confusing. Cholesterol is a non-water-soluble substance that does not move by itself through our blood. Instead, it is transported by *lipoproteins*. Lipoproteins are divided into three classes: high-density lipoproteins (HDLs), low-density lipoproteins (LDLs), and very-low-density lipoproteins (VLDLs). HDLs are sometimes called "good" cholesterol because they don't clog your blood vessels, and even seem to help your body cleanse itself of the "bad" cholesterol —the LDLs and VLDLs—which does clog your blood vessels and which may lead to stroke, heart attack, and peripheral vascular disease.

When you eat a great deal of saturated fats your body responds by manufacturing more LDLs and VLDLs—the "bad" cholesterol. However, polyunsaturated fats encourage the production of HDLs (the "good" cholesterol) and help lower the levels of VLDLs and LDLs. Unfortunately, for most people, 70 percent of the cholesterol in their blood is VLDLs or LDLs.

A healthy dietary goal would be to reduce overall fat consumption to a maximum of 30 percent of your daily calories. Your fat consumption should favor polyunsaturated fats over saturated fats. For most people, this means they need to reduce their saturated fat consumption while increasing their polyunsaturated fats. But do *not* overdo the polyunsaturated fats—remember, you should replace saturated fats with polyunsaturated fats within the context of a reduced total fat consumption diet and reduced calories.

STRATEGY
EATING LESS FAT

Try eating chicken, turkey, fish, or legumes and pasta as primary sources of animal protein. These foods contain less fat than most beef or pork. Remember to remove the skin from chicken and turkey before eating.

Eat less meat. Try instead rich sources of vegetable protein such as peas and beans. Currently, 70 percent of our protein consists of meat and dairy products, while many nutritionists suggest that only one-third of our protein should come from animals and two-thirds from vegetables. Meat and dairy products are major sources of saturated fats, while vegetables contain no cholesterol and little fat.

If you do eat beef, try to eat the leanest cuts possible and trim as much fat off as possible. Watch out for meat that is heavily marbled with white fat that runs through the cut. The "cheaper" cuts of meat are cheaper because they're tougher; they're tougher because they are *less* fatty and *better* for you.

Avoid meat with high fat or high cholesterol content, like bacon, ham, spareribs, sausage, salamis, duck, tongue, goose, hot dogs, canned meats, and organ meats like kidneys and liver.

Instead of frying meat, broil or roast it. This allows most of the fat to drip off.

Use low-fat or skim milk and milk products such as yogurt. Try reducing your servings of dairy products to one or two servings daily. Limit your consumption of hard or processed cheeses—they are loaded with fat and cholesterol. Learn which cheeses are low in fat.

When cooking, try not to use butter, lard, or solid vegetable shortenings; instead, use polyunsaturated vegetable oil and soft (not stick) margarine.

Read labels and ingredients lists and try to avoid foods that contain coconut oil, palm oil, hydrogenated fat or oil, or those that simply state "vegetable oil." These oils may be high in saturated fat content. After cooking soups, stews, or spaghetti sauce, chill them before eating. The saturated fats will float to the top and can easily be skimmed off.

Avoid chocolate (well, at least try to cut down—anything that tastes that good has got to be bad for you). Alas, most chocolates are loaded with saturated fats. Unfortunately, 70 percent of the calories in milk chocolate bars come from fat, not sugar!

HOT TOPIC #3: THE ANTICANCER DIET

Most experts agree that environmental factors such as diet and tobacco are involved in most human cancers. In fact, some estimates suggest that both diet and tobacco may each account for 30 percent or more of all cancers in the United States. While the link between smoking and cancer is clearly established, the relationship between diet and cancer is not precise. Our diet is a complex subject; it consists of many different types of foods and nutrients, with the possibility of tremendous variety within these food groups. For example, people who are in a low-risk cancer group may eat a lot of vitamin A, but they may also have a diet low in saturated fats. Which dietary factor—vitamin A or low saturated fats—is responsible for their low cancer risk? Furthermore, cancers may take many years and pass through different stages in development, all subject to different factors which may cause the cancer. Quite clearly, it is a difficult task, requiring many more years of study, to forge a direct link between dietary factors and cancer.

However, in spite of this difficulty, strong links between cancer and diet do exist. An impressively large body of studies conducted during the last few decades support the belief that some diets can increase the risk of cancer, while other diets may decrease the risk. Many studies have focused especially on the effects of vitamin A on cancer, in addition to vitamins C, E, and the trace metal selenium. Other studies have noted the relationship between a low-fiber, high-fat diet and cancer.

Vitamin A

Vitamin A, because it helps to foster healthy skin and mucous membranes, is thought to help prevent cancers found in the lung and bladder. A study at the State University of New York at Buffalo found that heavy smokers who consumed low levels of vitamin A were four times as likely to get cancer as those who ate high levels of vitamin A. Another study conducted over a nineteen-year period, involving 1,954 men, found that there was a significant relationship between a low vitamin A intake and a higher incidence of lung cancer, corresponding with a high vitamin A intake resulting in a lower cancer rate. The problem with these studies is the difficulty involved in accurately assessing a person's vitamin A intake, since the data is usually gathered through questionnaires and interviews. Nevertheless, the data in favor of vitamin A is impressive.

Other Nutrients

The effects of vitamins C and E, along with selenium (a trace metal found in seafood, garlic, whole grain cereals, and other sources), on cancer are currently being investigated in human studies. Exactly how these nutrients may assert an anticancer effect is still unclear.

All over the world, geographical areas with low selenium levels in the soil generally have higher cancer rates than areas with higher selenium levels. In one animal study involving rats on a cancer-producing diet, animals given selenium had fewer liver tumors than those given sorbic acid (a preservative) or nothing at all. Furthermore, rats given the most selenium for the longest period of time had the fewest tumors overall. In general, a large number of laboratory and animal studies support the belief that increased intake of selenium may reduce the incidence of cancer in humans.

Vitamin C, taken in very large doses, is currently being studied as a weapon against the creation of cancer-causing agents in the digestive tract. Researchers have reported that large doses of vitamin C has successfully treated a precancerous condition called familial polyposis, which eventually leads to cancer of the colon or rectum. *However,* other studies involving vitamin C as an anticancer agent have proven inconclusive. One article in *The New England Journal of Medicine* states "there is little empirical evidence that vitamin C provides protection against cancer in human beings" (3/8/84, p. 637, Drs. W. C. Willet and B. MacMahon).

Another animal study involving mice with colon/rectal tumors and vitamin E found that high doses of vitamin E significantly reduced the number of tumors. However, this antitumor effect has not been observed consistently.

Clearly, more research is warranted regarding the effects of these vitamins and nutrients on cancer in human subjects. It is strongly recommended that you refrain from arbitrarily taking massive doses of any vitamin—megadoses of vitamins can lead to serious and toxic effects. Please discuss any major diet change with your doctor prior to trying it out on yourself.

Fiber and Cancer

Colon/rectal cancer occurs most frequently in Western countries. In fact, Western countries (which consume a low-fiber diet) have a colon cancer rate *eight times greater* than many developing countries (which usually have high-fiber diets). These statistics have led many doctors to conclude that there is a link between fiber consumption and cancer. This may be an oversimplification, since the differences between developed and industrialized countries are complex, and include other dietary factors, such as meat and fat consumption. The situation gets even more confusing when you consider that many high-fiber foods may also contain other vitamins and nutrients that may have an anti-cancer effect.

Nevertheless, the weight of existing data supports the connection between a high-fiber diet (including high-fiber foods such as fruits and vegetables) and a lower risk of colon cancer. (For more information regarding fiber and your diet, see pages 167–171.)

Dietary Fat and Colon Cancer

Some evidence exists showing a link between a diet high in fat and an increased risk of colon cancer. In Japan, marked increases in rates of colon cancer have been associated with recent increases in fat intake. However, other studies have failed to find any association. At this time, more studies are needed to clearly establish a connection between dietary fat and colon cancer.

Dietary Fat and Breast Cancer

Many Asian and underdeveloped countries have rates of breast cancer that are as low as one-fifth that of the United States and northern Europe. Interestingly, children of Japanese immigrants, but *not* the immigrants themselves, have rates of breast cancer similar to the general American population. The statistics involving increased national consumption of fat and increased rates of breast cancer, have lead many doctors to postulate that there is a connection between the two. However, other population studies have failed to reinforce this position. At this point, there seems to be enough evidence to support the belief that at least some forms of dietary fat may cause breast cancer. And yet this position is far from being proved. Once again, more studies are needed. However, please note reduced dietary fat consumption provides many significant health benefits. (For more information on fat and your diet, see Chapter Six.)

HOT TOPIC #4: DIETS THAT WON'T BEAT THE ODDS

As stated elsewhere in this book (see Chapter Six), the only safe and effective way to lose weight is to eat less while maintaining a properly balanced diet—and exercise more. There is no mystical secret to losing weight. And yet, each year millions of Americans fork over millions of dollars on diet books and plans that promise to help the dieter lose weight with little or no effort. Unfortunately, some of these popular weight-loss programs may cause serious—even fatal—side effects. This section will look at some of these popular plans, along with some of the problems they may cause. The key, of course, with any diet is to consult your doctor before you embark on a particular program. It is important to realize that the diets discussed below can be perfectly fine for some people. But it is just as important to realize that they can be harmful to others.

Carbohydrate-Restricted Diets

With the introduction of the Atkins diet in 1972, low-carbohydrate diets became popular. The Atkins diet restricts carbohydrate intake to less than 40 grams per day, while allowing for unlimited protein and fat consumption. Some other low-carbohydrate diets are the Stillman diet, the Scarsdale diet, and the Drinking Man's diet. During the first week of these diets, there is an exaggerated water loss that is not fat loss. This allows claims of greater weight loss than actually happens.

These diets can be dangerous because they are high in fat content. They can produce high blood levels of uric acid, and may lead to an attack of gouty arthritis. These diets may also raise blood levels of cholesterol, thereby leading to an increased risk of heart attack and stroke. Also, the excessive proteins present in these diets may place an extra strain on your kidneys.

These low-carbohydrate diets may also promote the production of ketones, which in turn may lead to a condition called ketosis. Ketosis can cause nausea, vomiting, fatigue, and low blood pressure, and is especially harmful to pregnant women. In addition, the Atkins and Stillman diets are both deficient in niacin, iron, thiamine, riboflavin, and calcium.

The Beverly Hills Diet

The author of *The Beverly Hills Diet* claims that "Being fat has nothing to do with what you eat or how much you eat, but rather with the combination of foods you eat." This diet proposes that you should consume only carbohydrates with carbohydrates, protein with protein or fat, fruits by themselves, and fat with protein or carbohydrates. As one doctor, in the trade magazine *Drug Therapy,* has written: "None of these statements has any currently accepted physiological basis."

This diet may cause fluid and electrolyte depletion, along with low blood pressure. The Beverly Hills diet is also estimated to be deficient in the amounts of iron, vitamin D, phosphorus, and riboflavin it provides.

Liquid-Protein Diets

These protein-sparing diets require almost total fasting—with the only nourishment being a liquid-protein preparation. These diets were originally intended to help extremely obese people lose large amounts of weight (i.e., 100 pounds) under *strict medical supervision only*. Unfortunately, many people began following these diets with no medical supervision—often with tragic results. People following a protein-sparing diet *must* be monitored closely by medical personnel experienced in treating patients on very-low-calorie diets.

Many of the liquid protein dietary supplements purchased in drugstores are designed to *supplement,* not *replace,* a regular diet. This is true also for a protein-sparing diet. In the opinion of the general medical community, these diets remain experimental, although they have some promise when used in a multidisciplinary setting of medical supervision, modified fasting, behavior therapy, and exercise.

The following charts provide a comparison of some of the most

COMPARISON OF DIETS TO DIETARY GOALS

(Percent distribution of energy sources)

		▨ % PROTEIN	☐ % FAT	☐ % CARBOHYDRATE
DIETARY GOALS		15	30	55

DIETS	**CALORIES**	% PROTEIN	% FAT	% CARBOHYDRATE
Beverly Hills	928	6	4	90
F-Diet	1241	18	20	62
Pritikin 1200	1273	24	9	66
Pritikin 700	737	30	10	60
I ♥ America	1307	24	29	46
Simmons	924	26	29	45
I ♥ New York	980	32	30	38
Scarsdale	1014	28	31	41
Atkins	2031	23	73	4
Stillman	1316	46	49	5

0%   25%   50%   75%   100%

Data compiled by Dr. Paul A. La Chance, and
Michelle C. Fisher, R.D., Rutgers University, 1983.

VITAMIN AND MINERAL CONTENT OF TEN POPULAR REDUCING DIETS

		AVERAGE DAILY CALORIES	VITAMIN A	VITAMIN C	THIAMINE	RIBOFLAVIN	NIACIN	VITAMIN B6	FOLACIN	VITAMIN B12	CALCIUM	IRON	PHOSPHORUS	ZINC	MAGNESIUM
Pritikin 700	LOW	737	325	786	69	98	88	79	157	35	82	77	91	49	79
Simmons		924	70	165	64	83	105	50	56	51	60	42	87	40	53
Beverly Hills		928	461	798	56	50	40	96	405	0	34	50	27	32	69
I ♥ New York		980	386	551	60	125	126	73	106	291	82	92	118	74	102
Scarsdale	CALORIES	1014	222	555	57	71	115	65	84	37	51	55	90	74	52
F-Diet		1241	291	317	153	171	175	140	283	48	89	144	180	135	168
Pritikin 1200		1273	511	928	110	136	118	114	196	42	112	109	138	80	121
I ♥ America		1307	197	403	91	106	110	60	90	56	100	70	135	77	78
Stillman		1316	52	34	36	92	181	64	32	764	47	83	151	118	66
Atkins	HIGH	2031	92	92	70	94	107	67	64	110	88	64	144	87	48

Data compiled by Dr. Paul A. La Chance, and
Michelle C. Fisher, R.D., Rutgers University, 1983.

Percent of U.S. RDA
▨ Less than 70%
☐ 70–99%
☐ 100% or more

popular diet plans in relation to established dietary goals and Recommended Dietary Allowances of vitamins and minerals.

HOT TOPIC #5: CAFFEINE

The issue of whether caffeine contributes to heart disease and cancer has recently surfaced. Currently, there is conflicting data over caffeine and heart disease. It appears that caffeine consumption—in the form of coffee drinking—does not increase your chance of heart disease, unless coffee drinking exceeds five cups of caffeinated coffee daily. Less than five cups appears to have no effect on your risk of heart disease. My own advice is to drink two cups or less of caffeinated coffee daily. Better yet, use water extracted, decaffeinated coffee and avoid the issue altogether.

Caffeine and its relationship to cancer is even more confusing. There is conflicting evidence as to whether or not caffeine contributes to breast engorgement and nodularity (some experts believe this is a precancerous condition). Conversely, an early report suggests that cancer of the pancreas occurred more often if you drank decaffeinated coffee. Subsequent studies have shown a weak correlation between both caffeinated and decaffeinated coffee and pancreatic cancer.

In short, there is no link between cardiovascular disease and caffeine consumed in moderation. The issue of caffeinated coffee versus decaffeinated coffee as a risk for cancer has yet to be resolved.

Cancer

HOW YOUR DOCTOR DIAGNOSES CANCER

The confirmatory diagnosis of any sort of cancer usually depends on a biopsy: the removal from the body of a tissue specimen, which is then examined under a microscope by a pathologist. Examining the cellular structure of the tissue specimen, the pathologist determines whether or not the cell behavior in effect is abnormal and consistent with that observed in other malignant tissue. Cancer cells do not behave in an orderly manner; they exhibit bizarre behavior, as well as bizarre structures, when examined under a microscope. (See the box on page 182 for a list of cancer screening tests.)

LUNG CANCER

Lung cancer is often signaled by a worsening cough in a smoker, the presence of blood in the sputum, or by unusual, unexplained weight loss. Unfortunately for many patients, these symptoms don't bring them to the doctor until the disease is well advanced.

To diagnose lung cancer we X-ray the chest, check the sputum under a microscope to look for abnormal cells, and obtain a specimen

Periodic Examinations for Cancer Detection

Cancer detection is, of necessity, a procedure designed for the individual patient, not a mass screening effort. It may be prudent to modify these 1980 recommendations of the American Cancer Society ★ for individual patients.

TEST	PATIENT AGE	FREQUENCY
Breast physical examination	20–40	Every 3 years
	Over 40	Annually
Breast self-examination	Over 20	Monthly
Chest X ray	No specific recommendation	No specific recommendation
Digital rectal examination	Over 40	Annually
Endometrial tissue examination	At menopause ★★	
Mammography	35–40	One baseline
	40–49 ★★★	Every 1–2 years
	Over 50	Annually
Pap smear	20–65 and sexually active teenagers	2 consecutive years, then every 3 years
	At menopause	
Pelvic examination	20–40	Every 3 years
	Over 40	Annually
	At menopause	
Sigmoidoscopy	Over 50	2 consecutive years, then every 3–5 years
Sputum cytology	No specific recommendation	No specific recommendation
Stool guaiac	Over 50	Annually

★ ACS report on the cancer-related health checkup, *Ca* 1980, 30:194–240.
★★ For patients at high risk for endometrial cancer: obese women and those with a history of involuntary infertility, failure of ovulation, abnormal uterine bleeding, or estrogen therapy.
★★★ Revised 1983 recommendation.

of tissue from the lung by use of an instrument called a bronchoscope. This is a flexible tube that is passed down through the airways into the lung; a small tweezer passed through the tube is used to obtain a specimen of the lung tissue suspected of being malignant.

In breast cancer, as in most other cancers (not lung cancer, however) diagnosis is made by obtaining a specimen of the suspect tissue. Therefore, when a woman has a lump in her breast, and it is a firm, discrete nodule that a physician thinks may be abnormal, she will be advised to have a biopsy performed so that a pathologist can examine the cell histology. (See Chapter Fourteen for more information on breast cancer.)

COLON CANCER

The symptoms that may possibly indicate colon or rectal cancer include a marked change in bowel habits, often with intermittent constipation and loose bowel movements, or bleeding or blood within the bowel movement. Some colon cancers become evident because of pain in the lower abdomen, and some, particularly those in the right side of the colon, show evidence of anemia. To diagnose this cancer a specimen of the tumor is required; the most common procedure used to do this is a *colonoscopy,* a test in which a flexible lighted tube is inserted through the rectum to observe the lining mucosa of the colon and, ultimately, obtain tissue specimens for a biopsy. Prior to a colonoscopy, a series of X rays of the large intestine may be undertaken, utilizing a barium enema.

SKIN CANCER

Skin cancers usually have very few symptoms, and since they are the most accessible of all cancers, they can be detected readily by examination of any unusual growth or sore on the skin. They rarely cause death, since they tend not to be aggressive or invasive tumors. The majority of skin cancers are a form of *basal cell carcinoma.* On the other hand, *melanoma,* which arises from melanocytes, the cells that cause pigmentation in the skin, can spread to other organs and be fatal. Melanoma is the most serious skin cancer. Again, diagnosis is made by examination of the suspicious skin lesion.

LEUKEMIA

The *leukemias* usually appear in one of two ways. Either they are found on a routine examination, having caused no symptoms at all, or they are suspected because of lethargy or rapid onset of weight loss. Severe infections or easy bruising may also bring a patient to a physician and, ultimately, diagnosis. The diagnosis may simply require blood tests and an examination of a specimen of bone marrow, either from the chest or the hip.

SCREENING FOR CANCER

All these tests mentioned for the diagnosis of cancer can be performed as outpatient procedures, or during overnight or short-stay hospital admissions. However, once the initial diagnosis has been made, a longer hospital stay for more extensive investigation is often needed, to determine how advanced the tumor is.

In particular, it is important to determine whether the cancer is localized, contained within one small area in the lung, the breast, the colon, or the uterus, or whether the tumor has already metastasized (spread to other tissues). These determining tests may include, for example, the draining of lymph nodes near the breast, when the cancer may have spread to the lymph nodes in the axilla, or armpit. Likewise for the colon, it must be determined if the cancer cells have invaded through the muscular layer of the wall of the colon, or whether they have spread to the lymph nodes that drain the area of the colon that has cancerous lesions.

Screening for cancer means the regular use of diagnostic tests either to determine if a malignancy has developed, or if a precancerous lesion has appeared. In addition to having good tests that can diagnose the disease accurately in its early stages, we must be able to ensure that early diagnosis and treatment will result in the improvement of the overall survival of the patient. That is to say, if by diagnosing the cancer twelve months earlier we do not in fact increase the survival rate, then we are not gaining anything by undertaking regular examinations and checkups to see if cancer has developed. Unfortunately, lung cancer falls in this category. The possible screening tests include chest X rays and examination of sputum. Although chest X rays can be used in the diagnosis of lung cancer, they are not sensitive enough to diagnose lung cancer early and therefore prevent mortality. As mentioned before, stopping smoking and eliminating environmental factors really is the first and best step in preventing lung cancer.

For cancer of the colon and rectum, however, there is good evidence that regular examinations and testing can lead to early detection, and that early detection improves the survival rate substantially. The American Cancer Society recommends that all persons age 40 and over should have an annual digital rectal examination. A stool blood test to detect blood in the feces should be added to the annual exam at age 50.

In addition, *sigmoidoscopy*—an examination in which a small, lighted tube is passed into the rectum to examine the lining—should be performed every three to five years after age 50.

Furthermore, persons who are at high risk of developing colon or rectal cancer should receive more frequent and intensive examinations beginning at an earlier age. This includes people with family histories of polyps of the colon or cancer of the colon and rectum.

Cancer of the cervix (see Chapter Seventeen) accounts for about 4 percent of all cancers diagnosed in women in the United States. It has been shown to have survival rates that depend upon the stage at which the disease is detected. It, too, is ideally suited to the application of regular screening, and the Pap test has been in use for many years for this very purpose. This test takes a scraping of cells from the cervix, which can then be examined microscopically. The cell types indicating a precancerous lesion or a cancer can be seen with a microscope. It has been recommended that all women age 20 and over should have a Pap test annually for two negative exams, and then every three years until age 65.

A pelvic exam should be done as part of a general physical examination every three years from age 20 to age 40, and annually after age 40. We've also mentioned the association of endometrial cancer with estrogen use, and it's recommended that women who are at high risk of developing endometrial cancer (discuss your risk with your gynecologist) should have an annual Pap test, pelvic test, and an examination of endometrial tissue.

For breast cancer, for years the most frequent cancer in women, there is evidence that the probability of surviving the disease is increased with early detection. A recent study showed that for women who had their breast cancer diagnosed as a local disease, 85 percent survived at least five years, whereas for those who were diagnosed with the cancer already spread to lymph nodes, only 53 percent survived for five years.

Much of the evidence on the value of regular examinations for the early detection of breast cancer comes from a large study that was carried out by the Health Insurance Plan of Greater New York. This study, which began in 1964, examined the effects of annual physical examinations and mammograms on women, and the subsequent diagnosis, treatment, and survival rates of breast cancer. Although there is little objective information on the value of breast self-examinations, almost half of American women perform these exams on a monthly basis. Because early detection of breast cancer has been shown to decrease mortality, and since self-examination results in earlier detection, this procedure is definitely recommended; probably all women over 20 should perform breast self-examination monthly. In addition, women from 20 to 40 should have a breast physical examination every three years and women over 40 should have a breast physical examination every year. This reflects, in part, the increase in risk of breast cancer with increasing age.

Finally, based primarily on the results of the study from New York, it is recommended that women should have a baseline mammogram taken between ages 35 and 40; over age 50 they should have a mammogram every year. Women with higher risks of breast cancer due to family history should probably have some of these guidelines modified; since they are known to be at higher risk, they should have mammograms at an earlier age.

HOW YOU CAN HELP DETECT CANCER

Perhaps the most important initial approach to detecting cancer may be a thorough personal and family history evaluation conducted by your doctor. With this history, your doctor will determine if you have a special risk for developing cancer.

BREAST CANCER

The American Cancer Society (ACS) recommends that most women receive a breast examination conducted by their doctor *every three years* for women age 20 to 40, and *annually* for women over 40 years old. The ACS also recommends that a baseline mammogram be performed on women age 35 to 40, followed by mammography every one to two years for women age 40 to 49, and annually for women age 50 and over. The importance of a mammography should not be underestimated, even in women who have no cancer symptoms, since the National Cancer Institute estimates that 33 percent of all breast cancers occur in women 35 to 49 years old, and that most of these cancers were detected by mammography. Since many of these cancers were detected early—before the cancer had a chance to spread—there was a high potential for cure. Depending upon your family history or the presence of other risk factors for breast cancer (such as first pregnancy after age 25), your doctor may alter your schedule for breast examinations or mammography.

The ACS also recommends that women over 20 examine their breasts every month. Premenopausal women should examine their breasts one week after their menstrual period. Postmenopausal women should use the calendar to establish a monthly schedule.

Proper Techniques for Breast Self-Examination

Breast self-examination should begin in the shower, while standing upright. Your breast examination will be facilitated by thoroughly covering each breast with soap. Use the opposite hand to examine each breast (i.e., the right hand should examine the left breast and the left hand, the right breast). At least two fingers should be used, but avoid using the fingertips or fingernails, since the flat surface of the palmar pads (located on the top third of the palm side of each finger) are more sensitive. Usually the arm on the side being examined should be raised and placed on top of the head or neck. However, a very large breast may require support provided by the palm of the hand on the side being examined. It is *very important* to examine the entire breast area—from the collarbone to the armpits to just below each breast—since a lump may appear in any of these areas.

To ensure that every inch is covered, a systematic pattern of examination may be employed. The most popular method—developed by the American Cancer Society—involves a pattern of concentric circles. Begin at the outermost perimeter of the breast and, while gently pressing down on the skin, complete one full circle. Then move in approximately two finger widths and repeat the process. Notice that as you get closer to the nipple and areola area, the skin becomes more slippery and granular. Be very careful to feel for underlying lumps when examining these areas.

After completing this initial examination, you should proceed immediately to the second step. While standing, support one breast with a hand, then use the other hand to examine the top half of the breast, making small, circular movements with your fingers. When you have finished examining the top half, hold the top hand firmly against the breast and use the hand on the underside of the breast to search for lumps in the lower half. Repeat this process for the other breast.

The third step takes place while lying on your back. You may find it helpful to place a thin piece of cloth over your breasts—the thin material facilitates the immobilization of the skin while the fingers move. Try to keep the breast from falling to either side—raising your right shoulder with a pillow will help to keep the right breast centered correctly (and keep the left shoulder raised for the left breast). The arm on the side being examined should be placed behind your head. Now use the circular pattern explained above to examine the breast. Repeat this process with the arm on the side being examined resting alongside your body. Repeat the procedure for the other breast. If you find any lumps, or even if you *think* you may have found a lump, notify your physician *immediately*. This may turn out to be a false alarm, but that is a decision only your doctor should make.

DETECTING GYNECOLOGIC CANCERS

As we've said, the American Cancer Society (ACS) recommends that sexually active teenagers and women 20 to 65 years old receive a Pap smear first two consecutive years, followed by a Pap smear every three years. However, many gynecologists recommend annual Pap smears.

As we also mentioned earlier, the ACS recommends a pelvic examination every three years for women age 20 to 40, and yearly examinations for women over 40 years old. And don't forget that many gynecologists feel that a yearly pelvic examination is indicated for all women whose ovaries are intact, and annual examinations may even be necessary for women who have had their ovaries removed. Other uterine tissue examinations may also be in order. (See Chapter Nineteen for more information on this subject.)

The frequency of these tests may vary depending upon the presence of other risk factors. Obese women, especially if they also have diabetes, are more likely to get uterine cancer. Women with histories of infertility and failure to ovulate are also more likely to suffer uterine cancer. And women undergoing long-term estrogen therapy—without concomitant progesterone therapy—have a higher risk of getting uterine cancer. Cervical cancer appears more often in women who are sexually active at an early age. In addition, cervical cancer occurs more often in obese women. These are some of the risk factors that your doctor must know about to determine the type and frequency of your examinations.

Women should inform their doctor of any unusual bleeding (including bleeding after sex), painful sexual intercourse, or increasing abdominal growth. These symptoms may reflect the presence of a malignant growth and should be brought to your doctor's attention immediately.

CANCER RISK FACTORS AND SELF-DETECTION IN MEN AND WOMEN

Screening for lung cancer is directly connected to the presence of specific risk factors: whether or not you smoke cigarettes, how long you have smoked, the number of cigarettes you smoke each day, and whether you work or have worked in an industry where air pollution (e.g., asbestos) is present. These determine if you are at heightened risk for lung cancer. Interestingly, a family history of lung cancer probably does not increase your chances of developing lung cancer; rather, it is your own cigarette smoking and/or exposure to environmental factors that may place you at a special risk.

Symptoms that may indicate lung cancer include a persistent cough, a radical change in the type of cough, coughing up blood, and pneumonia that affects one or more of the lobes of the lungs. If you experience any of these symptoms, your doctor may recommend a chest X ray and an analysis of your sputum (the mucus you expectorate).

COLON/RECTAL CANCER

People with a high risk of developing colon/rectal cancer include those with a history of ulcerative colitis, adenomatous polyps (small polypoid tumors in the colon), multiple polyps, and a family history of colon/rectal cancer or intestinal polyps.

For people with no symptoms and who have no special risk of developing colon/cancer, the American Cancer Society (ACS) recommends annual digital rectal examination for people over 40 years old. Also, for people over age 50, the ACS suggests an annual stool guaiac test, to detect the presence of blood. Many gynecologists prefer to use the stool guaiac test on three successive stools. The ACS suggests that a sigmoidoscopy (which provides a more "in depth" examination than just a digital rectal examination) be performed for people over 50 years old.

Colon/rectal cancer may be indicated by the presence of blood in the stool, a change in bowel habits, anemia, or prolonged stomach pain. If you experience any of these symptoms, you should notify your doctor.

TESTICULAR CANCER

Each year, about 4,000 American men develop cancer of the testes. Testicular cancer strikes men most often between the ages of 20 and 40, although it can occur at any age. As with many other forms of cancer, early detection of testicular cancer dramatically increases the chances of a cure. In fact, this form of cancer is perhaps the most easily cured form—when detected early. However, when detected late, testicular cancer may be fatal. Unfortunately, almost 50 percent of cases are detected *after* the cancer has spread.

Doctors as well as patients are frequently responsible for the delay in diagnosis. Men hesitate in reporting any growths or abnormalities in their testes because they fear treatment will render them impotent. (Only in very rare cases will early detection and treatment of testicular cancer result in impotence.) And even when doctors notice a recognizable abnormality in the testes, they are reluctant to perform a key diagnostic test, the removal of the testes for examination. Although other tests may aid in diagnosing testicular cancer, the most successful examination involves removal of a testes. The removal of a single testes usually does not result in sterility—and it may prove essential in detecting cancer.

Self-Examination of the Testes

The chance for early detection is enhanced greatly when a man examines his testes on a regular basis. Some types of testicular cancer grow very rapidly—the loss of even one or two months in diagnosing

Know the Seven Warning Signs of Cancer

C-A-U-T-I-O-N

Change in bowel or bladder habits
A sore that does not heal
Unusual bleeding or discharge
Thickening or lump in breast or elsewhere
Indigestion, difficulty in swallowing
Obvious change in wart or mole
Nagging cough or hoarseness
If you have a warning signal, see your doctor immediately.

these may prove very costly. Many doctors urge men to examine their testes every month.

The best time to examine your testes is during or after a warm bath or shower. A healthy testes is smooth and free of lumps, except for the soft, tubelike lump along the back, where sperm is stored. When examining your testes you should apply a small amount of pressure with the thumb and fingers of both hands to each testes. Most abnormalities are not attached to the scrotum (the sac containing the testes) and are usually found along the front or side of the testes. Any abnormalities that you find, or even think you have found, should be reported immediately to your doctor.

Remember, early detection is the most important action involved in curing most cancers. The more responsibility you take in examining yourself, the greater your chances of beating the cancer odds.

OTHER CANCER RISK FACTORS

As you know, not all smokers get lung cancer, and so you may ask what factors influence a person's susceptibility to the development of a cancer. Several factors have been identified by scientific studies. The incidence or onset of cancer in general is related to age; as people get older, their risk of getting cancer is higher.

Family History

You may have also heard that cancer runs in families. Certainly there are some cancer types that are more likely among relatives than as compared to the general population. The cancers that have this familial association include breast cancer, gastric (stomach) cancer, and some forms of colon cancer. In addition, there is a small familial or genetic contribution to cancer of the uterus. For colon cancer, there is a three- to four-fold higher risk for the disease in relatives of patients than in the general population. In addition, many of the disorders of the colon that predispose people to developing cancer, including familial colonic polyps, are inherited. The familial association for breast cancer is strongest for women developing breast cancer before menopause. The small familial component of the risk of uterine cancer appears to be related to several of the disorders of ovarian function that are themselves inherited. These disorders of ovarian function and hormone secretion lead to relative infertility, which increases the risk of uterine cancer.

Diet

Another factor that may modify a person's susceptibility to cancer is diet. The wide variation from nation to nation in incidence rates for cancers of specific sites suggests a possible association with diet for several cancers. In particular, there has been much study of the effects of diet on modifying the risk of lung cancer in smokers, of the effects of fat and fiber intake on risks of breast cancer, and on colon cancer.

Given the biochemical behavior of several of the nutrients obtained from vegetables and other foods, it is possible that these nutrients reduce the natural damaging processes that go on in the body and also reduce the damage caused by external agents such as cigarette smoke or ultraviolet light. Several studies have shown that smokers who consume a diet with a high content of certain vegetables (including dark green, leafy vegetables such as spinach, yellow vegetables such as carrots and squash, and also including broccoli and brussel sprouts), have less than half the risk of developing lung cancer compared to smokers who have a low intake of these vegetables. Of course, these people could reduce their risk much more by stopping smoking than by changing their diet.

Smoking

Tobacco is probably the greatest contributor to the incidence of cancer in the United States today that can be clearly avoided. People who smoke have a ten times greater chance of developing cancer than people who don't smoke. In particular, the most obvious association between smoking and cancer is that almost ALL lung cancer is associated with smoking. Smoking is associated with 30 percent of all cancer deaths in the United States.

The risk of getting lung cancer increases with the number of years that a person smokes. In addition, the younger a person is when he or she starts smoking, the greater the risk of developing lung cancer. Smoking has also been linked to cancers of the larynx, esophagus, and mouth, as well as cancer of the kidney and the bladder.

Recent confirmation of the evidence that smoking is related to lung cancer includes the steady rise of lung cancer incidence in women in the United States, a rise that parallels the increasing number of women who smoke. It is expected that within the next ten years more women will die from lung cancer than from breast cancer. When a smoker stops smoking, the risk of lung cancer takes quite some time to return to the level of the nonsmoker. For someone who has been a heavy smoker for a long time, it takes up to ten years for the risk of lung cancer to return to the risk of someone who has never smoked.

Ionizing Radiation

Ionizing radiation is one of the most extensively studied causes of cancer in humans. Almost all human cancers can be induced by radiation if the exposure is great enough. Some of the evidence for this comes from the followup studies of people exposed to the atomic bomb in Japan. The greatest source of exposure to ionizing radiation for the general population comes from natural background sources. These include cosmic rays and radiation from the ground. The greatest manmade source is the medical X ray. The study of people with diseases that had to be treated by X ray—including ankylosing spondylitis treatment and outdated therapy modes for tuberculosis—has shown that being exposed to regular high doses of X rays increases the risk for developing cancer.

Solar Radiation

Solar radiation, or sun exposure, has been clearly linked as the primary risk factor for skin cancer. Skin cancer is predominantly a disease of the white race, and especially common in fair-complexioned individuals who tend to sunburn. These people are notably of Irish,

Scottish, Welsh, and Scandinavian backgrounds. Furthermore, it occurs primarily on parts of the body with direct exposure to sunlight. Those areas of the body that receive the highest chronic doses of ultraviolet exposure are those that develop skin cancers. The damage to the skin caused by sun exposure can readily be avoided by the wearing of protective clothing and the application of sunscreen lotions designed to prevent the penetration of ultraviolet rays from the sun.

Alcohol

Alcohol has been most convincingly associated with cancers of the gastrointestinal tract. Several studies have shown the fact that alcohol increases the risk for oral and esophageal cancer even in nonsmokers —and also that alcohol and, in particular, beer are associated with increased risk of rectal cancer. Finally, in people who develop alcoholic liver disease, the risk of primary liver cancer is greatly increased.

Other conditions that cause cirrhosis of the liver, such as chronic hepatitis, likewise increase the risk of primary liver cancer. However, alcohol again is an identifiable, preventable cause.

Viruses

The investigation of viruses as a cause of cancer has been in progress for many years. To date it is suggested that the viruses are associated with African Burkitt's lymphoma, a tumor that has a high incidence in children in Africa and in other tropical areas. There is also evidence of possible viral involvement in leukemia and Hodgkin's disease. In addition, there has been much focus on the possible role of herpes simplex virus in the etiology of cervical cancer. However, at present the evidence is not convincing.

Drugs

The association between drugs and cancer refers primarily to endometrial cancer. The use of estrogen supplements for women after menopause has been clearly shown to be associated with the risk of endometrial cancer. In the absence of exogenous estrogens, the incidence rate of endometrial cancer is approximately 1 per 1,000 postmenopausal women per year. This rate increases severalfold after a woman commences using estrogen. The risk of endometrial cancer increases with the duration of use of estrogen replacement therapy and declines after discontinuation of estrogen. (See Chapter Seventeen for more information.)

Although estrogen replacement therapy has been associated with uterine cancer, there is no suggestion of any association with breast cancer, and no adverse effects when estrogens are used for the prevention of osteoporosis. Cycling estrogen with progesterone should provide protection against osteoporosis and symptoms of menopause without increasing the risk of endometrial cancer.

Other sex hormones that women may be exposed to include oral contraceptives, for which there is, to date, no evidence of an association with breast cancer. In the past, some women were exposed to DES (diethylstylbestrol), which has been associated with a rare form of vaginal cancer in the *daughters* of women who had used this drug during pregnancy.

TREATMENT OF CANCER

The primary aim in the treatment of cancer is to remove cancerous tissue by surgical excision. This is most effective when the cancer is confined to one site or is a primary lesion. If at the time of diagnosis the cancer has already spread to other sites, then the probability of long-term survival for the patient is considerably reduced.

In addition to surgical removal of cancerous tissue, many treatment programs include both radiation therapy, either to the cancer site and the draining lymph nodes or to the appropriate lymphatic region of the body, and the use of chemotherapeutic drugs. In effect, these drugs kill the most rapidly dividing cells in the body. Since it is cancer cells that are the most rapidly dividing cells in the body, they are most susceptible to these drugs and, hopefully, can be eliminated from the body by the administration of the appropriate combination of drugs.

The site of the cancer being treated and the cancer's cellular structure determines in large part which drugs should be used for chemotherapy. The effectiveness of both radiation therapy and chemotherapy have continued to improve over the past ten years, but the early detection of a cancer and its surgical removal prior to extensive growth and metastasis by the tumor remains the best form of treatment. With improved techniques of administering radiotherapy and chemotherapy, the side effects and deformities that have frightened people in the past have been greatly minimized.

Of course, if we could avoid agents that cause cancer, such as cigarettes and other risk factors, then we would be avoiding the whole need to diagnose and treat the cancer. For instance, knowing that a loved one has recently been diagnosed as having lung cancer, you may well wonder what you can do to reduce the risk of your developing cancer yourself. Stopping smoking certainly would be the first and most important strategy. In addition, there might be other steps that you should probably be taking to reduce the risk of developing cancer, such as awareness of environmental factors and, alternatively, promoting an early diagnosis should you be unlucky enough to develop it. Contact your local Cancer Society or Lung Association to find out what may be contaminating the air you breathe at work.

Cancer Is Curable

Early detection and treatment increase the probability of survival— that is, decrease the long-term effects of the cancer once treatment is initiated. This is true for most cancers.

Different strategies for the prevention of cancer can be found in Beating the Smoking Odds (Chapter Nine), Beating Alcohol and Drug Abuse Odds (Chapter Ten), and General Diet Tips to Beat the Odds (Chapter Twelve).

Respiratory Diseases

THE COMMON COLD

The common cold, also known as upper respiratory tract infection, is perhaps the most common of all diseases. This is the usual head cold or chest cold with which we are all so familiar from constant firsthand experience. Colds are almost always caused by viral infections of the upper respiratory tract. Because there are so many different families of viruses that can cause these illnesses, and because each virus family has so many members, there is a seemingly infinite variety of different viruses that can cause colds, against which we will never be able to develop universal immunity.

When the virus causes inflammation in the nose, we experience it as a stuffy nose (*coryza*) or as a runny nose (*rhinitis*), sometimes with postnasal drip. When inflammation involves the pharynx, we experience a sore throat and call it *pharyngitis*. If inflammation extends to the vocal cords, hoarseness or loss of voice (*laryngitis*) is the result. If the trachea and main bronchi are involved, symptoms of cough and chest congestion result, and sputum may be produced; this is referred to medically as a *tracheobronchitis* or *acute bronchitis*.

The diagnosis is usually made as easily by the patient as by the physician. Laboratory tests are rarely used because we are not skilled at isolating particular viruses that might be causing the infection, nor are specific treatments available should we be able to identify the virus.

INFLUENZA

Influenza is a virus that affects the respiratory tract in a particularly virulent way. It commonly causes severe aching in the muscles and joints, and prostration. Influenza spreads through communities in epidemic form and may cause very serious disease and even death, because it may lead to viral pneumonia (an infection of the lower respiratory tract) or, more commonly, because it predisposes the patient to bacterial pneumonia as a complication of the influenza infection. Influenza can be prevented by the use of the influenza vaccine. Because the influenza virus changes its makeup each year by mutation, a different vaccine must be given annually. It should be noted that the influenza virus is only one of a multitude of viruses that cause respiratory tract infections, so that if you develop a cold after receiving an influenza vaccine, it is not a reflection of a failure of that vaccine, nor is it necessarily caused by the vaccine even if it occurs immediately after vaccination.

PNEUMONIA

Pneumonia is different from viral upper respiratory tract infections in that it involves the very substance of the lung, the air spaces, or alveoli. Pneumonia is an infection of the lower respiratory tract, and it is particularly serious because it may interfere with the lungs' function in exchanging oxygen and carbon dioxide between the air and the blood. Common symptoms of pneumonia are fever, cough, and sputum production, which may in some cases be minimal and off-white in color; in other cases, the sputum may be yellow, green, or brown, and plentiful. Also, in some cases of pneumonia there is shortness of breath.

If pneumonia is complicated with inflammation of the covering of the lung, *pleurisy* is the result. Pleurisy involves a characteristic chest pain that hurts with each inspiration and causes the patient to take short, shallow breaths. Pneumonias may be caused by viruses, bacteria, or by intermediate forms called mycoplasma. If pneumonia is left untreated, very serious complications can develop; it becomes a life-threatening illness that can leave the lungs permanently damaged. However, treatment makes pneumonia a benign illness in most cases.

Drawing the distinction between pneumonia and a simple head and chest cold is not always easy, but the possibility of pneumonia should be considered when one has a fever in excess of 102 degrees—particularly if associated with shaking, teeth-rattling chills. Further symptoms include a cough that is productive of more than just a fraction of a teaspoon of thick, discolored sputum, a cough or sputum production that lingers beyond the usual time frame of a common cold, or the development of pleurisy or significant shortness of breath. It may not be possible for your physician to determine whether or not you have pneumonia simply by talking to you over the telephone. By examining your lungs, your physician may hear sounds that suggest disease involving the substance of the lung itself, and in some cases it may be necessary to obtain a chest X ray.

In a head or chest cold involving just the air tubes, the chest X ray would look normal, whereas in pneumonia, inflammation of the substance of the lung shows up on the X ray as an abnormality commonly referred to as an *infiltrate*. In diagnosing pneumonia, your physician may also wish to examine the sputum in order to identify the particular bacterium that may be causing this pneumonia. This is called a sputum gram stain and culture.

Some people seem to develop recurrent chest infections and pneumonias. Both heavy cigarette smoking and heavy alcohol consumption appear to interfere with your body's ability to fight respiratory infections and may predispose you to pneumonia.

Persons with underlying respiratory diseases, particularly chronic bronchitis and emphysema, have lungs that have an impaired ability to fight infections. In rare cases, there are immunologic diseases that disturb the body's natural defenses against infection. The importance of these defenses has become particularly apparent in the epidemic of acquired immune deficiency syndrome, or AIDS, a disease to which promiscuous male homosexuals and intravenous drug users are susceptible. The victims of AIDS often develop a particularly severe pneumonia called pneumocystis carinii pneumonia, as a result of the loss of function of one of the types of blood cells called "helper lymphocytes."

Pneumonia caused by mycoplasma or bacteria is treated with antibiotics. In the otherwise healthy individual who is not severely incapacitated by his or her illness, these antibiotics may be given on an outpatient basis. In those with underlying lung disease, or with more severe illness, the antibiotics are more properly given intravenously in the hospital. X rays should be followed until they show a complete clearing of the pneumonia with treatment.

The bacterium most often responsible for the pneumonia is the pneumococcus—hence the importance of the recent development of the pneumococcal vaccine. Anyone over the age of 60 or with a history of serious respiratory disease should be given the pneumococcal vaccine. This is particularly true of persons who have had their spleen removed or who have a spleen that does not function normally, as in sickle cell anemia, because the spleen is an important organ in fighting infections caused by the pneumococcus.

ASTHMA

Asthma is an exceedingly common disease in this country, affecting some 3 to 5 percent of the population at any given time. It is common in both young children and adults, and may develop at any age. Asthma is a disease characterized by an excessive sensitivity or irritability of the air tubes (bronchi) of the lung, so that a variety of stimuli that do not bother normal lungs will trigger an asthmatic narrowing and inflammation of those tubes.

What causes some people to have this condition of hyperreactive airways is unknown. Sometimes it develops in people with allergic diseases, particularly hay fever and eczema. In such patients with allergic predispositions, it would seem that asthma is a manifestation of allergy in their lungs. In others, no such allergic background is evident. Sometimes asthma seems to begin after a particularly serious viral upper respiratory tract infection, and at other times, no cause is evident.

In people who have this underlying tendency of abnormally irritable or reactive airways, a variety of stimuli will trigger an asthma attack. Such stimuli include inhaled allergens, such as pollen or mold, and inhaled irritants, such as cigarette smoke and smog. Exercise, particularly on a cold winter day, a head/chest cold, and, in some cases, emotional upset can also bring on an attack of asthma. A small percentage of asthmatics will be sensitive to aspirin, or to bisulfites, which are used as food preservatives in fresh fruits and vegetables, and in some wines. Some asthmatics react to tartrazine dye, a virtually ubiquitous food coloring, but this is fortunately quite unusual.

Symptoms of Asthma

Common symptoms of asthma are wheezing, cough, and shortness of breath, particularly with a sensation of tightness or congestion in the chest. What distinguishes this disease from the chronic lung diseases of emphysema and chronic bronchitis is that it is episodic. At times the lungs of an asthmatic are normal or near normal, and at times they may be quite severely abnormal, causing major respiratory distress. The disease is frequently diagnosed simply on the basis of the characteristic history of wheezing, cough, and shortness of breath on an episodic basis, usually related to the irritating substances mentioned earlier. At other times, diagnosis is confirmed with pulmonary function tests. These tests usually involve requiring a person to blow forcefully into machinery that records the size of the exhaled breath and the rate at which it is exhaled from the lungs. This type of test is commonly referred to as *spirometry*.

In some patients the diagnosis may not be quite so obvious. For instance, asthma may appear in some people simply as a persistent refractory cough. In others it may be indicated only by shortness of breath and chest tightness on exertion, which is called "exercise-induced asthma." In such persons, the pulmonary function test may be normal; only by stressing the respiratory system, by provoking narrowing of the air tubes (with one of the common stimuli, such as exercise), can one provoke an abnormal decrease in the flow of air from the lungs, thus bringing on the typical manifestation of asthma.

Problems with asthma are twofold. First, the involuntary muscle that rings the bronchial tubes can contract, narrowing those tubes and making it difficult for air to move in and out through them. This is called bronchospasm. The second problem is inflammation of the airways, or bronchi. This inflammation involves swelling, irritation, and secretion of mucus into the bronchial tubes, which further narrows them, making air movement difficult.

The treatment of asthma is then directed at these two abnormalities. One group of medicines are called bronchodilators. These medicines relax the muscle around the bronchial tubes, causing the tubes to dilate. Adrenaline and its relatives are bronchodilators, as are the family of drugs referred to as aminophylline or theophylline.

The second method of treatment of asthma uses antiinflammatory medications to reduce the inflammation in the airways. The strongest of these medicines are corticosteroids or steroids. (Cortisone and prednisone are examples of steroid medications.) A variety of bronchodilator medications are available over the counter; probably the best known of these is Primatene Mist. Also, a recent article suggested that two cups of coffee may have some weak bronchodilating effect.

The major problem with these medications is that they are not terribly effective. Primatene Mist is a relatively weak bronchodilator, one that gives relief for only a short period of time, and may have significant side effects in terms of stimulation of the heartbeat. If more effective medications are needed, they are available from your physician; these are more powerful, and are likely to have fewer side effects as well as longer-lasting benefits. In general, asthma is an ailment that the patient should self-medicate only within the guidelines set by a physician.

If you have asthma, it is important to minimize your exposure to stimuli that trigger attacks. The most sensible thing to do is to take a critical look at your immediate environment. Pets are often a source of animal dander. If it is not practical to get rid of a beloved cat or dog, at least it should be removed from your bedroom and kept out of doors or in the basement, if possible. After all you've read in this book, it should not be necessary to mention that cigarette smoking is a lunacy that should be immediately abandoned. Feather pillows can be replaced with synthetic-filled ones. Heavy dust-collecting shag rugs are best removed from the home. Most asthmatics, as they look about the home environment, are able to identify specific areas or items that repeatedly make them wheeze, and which they can then avoid.

This is also true about diet; a specific food that characteristically causes wheezing can be recognized and eliminated from the diet. Extensive skin testing by an allergist is not usually helpful and rarely provides useful information beyond what you can learn by examining your diet and your home environment by yourself. Also, in general, desensitization injections aimed at specific allergens do not seem effective in the treatment of asthma.

It is a common frustration for many asthmatics that their exercise capacity is limited, because frequently, when they do attempt to exercise, they begin to wheeze and develop tightness of the chest and shortness of breath. This is particularly true in cold weather, as cold, dry air brings on wheezing with even minimal exercise. Two measures can be taken to prevent this and to increase your ability to exercise. The first is to use your bronchodilator medicines prior to exercising. This is particularly effective with the inhaled medications and will help prevent the airway narrowing that would otherwise occur. The second is a simple technique to use on a cold winter day: Wear a scarf around your mouth and nose. In so doing, you can trap warm moist air in front of your mouth and decrease the amount of cold air that is inhaled deep into the lungs, air that would otherwise serve as a trigger stimulus to an asthma attack. So, you see, Grandmother was right—wear a scarf when you go out to play in winter.

Asthma is a common disease in women of childbearing age. In perhaps a quarter of asthmatics, the asthma will become worse during pregnancy. In others it seems not to change and sometimes even gets better. Although it is best to avoid all medications if possible during pregnancy, in general the medications that are used to treat asthma are safe. The low oxygen supply that may occur with a severe asthma attack is much more dangerous to the fetus. Do not avoid medical care of your asthma for fear of taking medicine that may harm the fetus; instead, seek medical care early in order to avoid significant asthma attacks, which are a more serious threat to the unborn child.

Finally, there are active asthma support groups, particularly for children with asthma. Lists of these are available through the American Lung Association, 1740 Broadway, New York, N.Y. 10019, (212) 315-8700; one of the better organizations is called Superbreath.

EMPHYSEMA AND CHRONIC BRONCHITIS

Emphysema and chronic bronchitis are diseases that are often spoken of together, lumped under the general heading of chronic obstructive pulmonary disease (COPD). They are often lumped together because they are the result of chronic inhalation of cigarette smoke, so both diseases are usually found to greater or lesser degrees in cigarette smokers. Both diseases would virtually be eliminated by the stopping of smoking. It is only in very rare cases of genetic disorder that emphysema appears as an inherited family trait that may occur even in nonsmoking family members.

Emphysema is destruction of the substance of the lung itself, in which there is loss of the elastic properties of the lung. This leads to difficulty in expelling air from the lungs, so that when the lungs are called upon to move air in and out quickly, they are unable to do so.

Chronic bronchitis is inflammation of the bronchial tubes, characterized by excess mucus production. The symptoms of chronic bronchitis are cough and sputum production. This begins as the typical smoker's cough, as in coughing and clearing the lungs of excess mucus each morning. One can diagnose chronic bronchitis by determining the presence of a cough with sputum production on a daily basis. Once it progresses, shortness of breath develops; this may show up in pulmonary function testing as decreased flow of exhaled air, much the same as in asthma. However, unlike asthma it is not episodic but permanent, and likely to be present more or less every day.

Emphysema is less easy to measure because we have no simple test to assess the elasticity or springiness of the lungs. As a result, we often rely on indirect evidence for emphysema—particularly a chest X ray that demonstrates excessively enlarged lungs with a reduction of the normal markings that are seen on the X ray. These X-ray findings, coupled with the characteristic limitation to the flow of air on exhalation found in pulmonary function testing (spirometry), may suggest the likelihood of emphysema in a heavy cigarette smoker.

TUBERCULOSIS

Tuberculosis, although far less common today than in years past, still occurs in thousands of persons each year. Misunderstandings cause a lot of confusion and fear about the disease. The fear is possibly due to the memory of tuberculosis when it was a disease called consumption and of the gradual wasting away of people afflicted by this disease. Also, people think of the tremendous personal hardship that used to be involved in treatment of the disease, by removal of the person with tuberculosis from the home environment to the sanitorium.

Things have changed enormously since the discovery that tuberculosis is caused by a type of infectious organism called a mycobacterium, very similar to the bacteria mentioned earlier in this chapter. Tuberculosis is an infection like other infections—it causes a pneumonia like other pneumonias—and in modern-day medicine it is treated with antibiotics just like other pneumonias. The treatment of tuberculosis is different from that of pneumonia in that usually at least two antibiotics are given concurrently, and the treatment must extend for a period of months, usually a minimum of nine months. This is because the mycobacterium that causes tuberculosis is very slow-growing and must be killed by using a prolonged course of treatment.

The symptoms of TB are essentially those of a chronic protracted pneumonia with fever, sweats at night, cough with discolored sputum production, weight loss, and perhaps shortness of breath. The diagnosis is suspected on the basis of an abnormality in the chest X ray and is confirmed by examination of the sputum that is expectorated. One acquires TB by inhaling the TB mycobacterium, which has been sprayed into the air by the coughing, speaking, or singing of someone with TB pneumonia.

Most people, if they inhale the mycobacterium, are able to fight off infection—to seal off the microorganism and never develop an illness. However, if tested for a TB infection with a skin test called a Tine test or PPD skin test, such people who inhaled the mycobacterium but never developed disease would develop a reaction in their skin, a positive skin test. It is important to realize that this is not evidence of TB pneumonia, simply evidence of having been exposed to the mycobacterium and having inhaled it into the lungs, successfully fighting off infection. The significance of such a positive test is that it confirms that you have the potential to develop TB at some point in your life, particularly if you develop a concurrent illness or some cause of debilitation.

This risk of someday developing TB can be prevented by taking a one-year course of medication of antituberculosis antibiotic. This one year of preventive antibiotic is strongly recommended for persons with a positive skin test who are young (less than 35 years of age), or who have acquired the positive skin test within the last two years, or who have been tested positively because of a strong exposure to a household member who has active TB disease.

To reiterate, a positive skin test for TB does not mean tuberculosis disease or tuberculosis pneumonia, but simply infection at some point in the past when the mycobacterium was inhaled. The chest X ray should be done to exclude the possibility of pneumonia, and in certain persons it is appropriate to prevent the future development of active TB disease with one year of antibiotic chemoprophylaxis (preventive treatment).

WHAT YOU CAN DO TO HELP REDUCE RESPIRATORY DISEASE RISK FACTORS

Basic Do's and Don'ts for Healthy Lungs

Probably the most important and overwhelming advice one can give for respiratory disease is, *don't smoke*. Or, if you already smoke, *quit smoking*. Cigarette smoking is the major cause of chronic respiratory illness in this country. Without cigarette smoking most cases of chronic bronchitis, emphysema, and lung cancer would simply disappear.

Smoking is very definitely an addiction—an extremely powerful psychological addiction as well as a chemical one to nicotine. The best way not to become addicted to cigarettes is never to start smoking. Many people suffocating on a daily basis, gasping for air with the least effort or exertion, have cursed their addiction to cigarettes, wishing that they had never started to smoke.

Other things that are most dangerous to inhale are generally found in the workplace. These are often inorganic fibers or dust, which when inhaled are deposited in the lungs, often causing chronic and generally untreatable lung disease. The best known of these fibers is asbestos. Exposure occurs to those working in the mining and manufacture of asbestos products, and to those who work with asbestos insulation in the construction industry or in the shipbuilding industry.

Auto mechanics may have recurrent exposure to asbestos when working with brake linings, and because for a time tile floors were lined with asbestos, those who were working in the floor-laying trades may have a problem in this area. Serious exposure generally takes place over a period of months to years, so that the occasional incident—for example, when you go into the basement and disturb a carefully wrapped asbestos-insulated pipe, breathing in a few dust particles on this one occasion—is not cause for alarm.

Other particles that are dangerous to inhale are silica, which one finds in the quarrying or sandblasting industries; beryllium, which was previously used in the manufacture of fluorescent lights and is now used in the aerospace industry; and coal dust, the well-known cause of black lung in coal miners. Attempts should be made to avoid these exposures; at times, even a change of job may be necessary. Take immediate steps to remedy the situation by contacting your local

Public Health agency. If you work in a dusty area or around fumes, wear a protective mask.

COMMON SYMPTOMS

One symptom that may signal serious respiratory disease is the appearance of a cough outside of the context of a common cold or chronic cigarette smoker's cough. Sputum production that is not caused by a head or chest cold and is not the typical smoker's hack should be called to the attention of your physician.

Shortness of breath is a subjective feeling that is experienced rather than measured. We all become short of breath with strenuous exertion, although what constitutes strenuous exertion will also vary from one person to another. If your exercise tolerance is limited by shortness of breath, or by lighter and lighter exercise levels over a relatively brief period of time, don't think this is simply growing older—particularly if you can no longer keep up with healthy companions of the same age.

Finally, coughing up blood is always abnormal, even in the setting of a chest cold. It should be explored as a possible early warning symptom of serious lung disease.

For general respiratory health, exercise is highly recommended. It cannot injure your lungs. If you become short of breath with exercise, you can simply rest and recover a normal sensation of breathing without permanent damage having been done. Exercise does not so much strengthen the lungs as it does the ability of the heart to pump blood. This increases the ability of your muscles in general to remove oxygen from the blood. Thus, a well-conditioned person can do the same level of work with less amount of respiratory stress than an unconditioned person. This is particularly to your advantage if the amount of breathing that you can do is limited by lung disease.

PREVENTIVE MEDICINE FOR THE RESPIRATORY SYSTEM

The influenza vaccine is available each winter for those over the age of 60 or with underlying respiratory conditions, and to those repeatedly exposed to ill persons in a health-care facility.

The most common type of bacterial pneumonia in adults is pneu-mococcal pneumonia, caused by the pneumococcus bacterium. A vac-cine is available that is 80 percent effective in protecting you from pneumonia caused by this bacterium. This pneumococcal vaccine should be given for the same indications as for the flu shot. However, unlike the flu shot, it is not to be given every year. The duration of protection from a single pneumococcal vaccine injection is currently unknown, but it is likely to be at least five or ten years, so that repeat vaccination with the pneumococcal vaccine is not currently recom-mended.

COMMON MISCONCEPTIONS ABOUT RESPIRATORY DISEASE

With the exception of very few persons suffering from asthma, *diet* does not make a major contribution to your respiratory health. If you suffer from respiratory illness, it is not because of what you have eaten, nor can you protect your good health by special diets. Perhaps the most controversial issue with respect to diet and respiratory health is the use of vitamin C to prevent or treat viral head colds. Although the use of vitamin C was proposed by a very famous scientist, all attempts at documenting its benefit scientifically have failed. It could be argued that if the use of vitamin C were effective in preventing the most common illness known to man, it would not be a secret known to just a few devotees but would rapidly become universally accepted and practiced; this is certainly not the case.

Another common misconception regarding respiratory disease is that it is important to learn the proper way to breathe. Physicians as well as respiratory therapists have spent many hours teaching patients with emphysema and chronic bronchitis the proper techniques of breathing. But since breathing is an unconscious act, this is a highly futile endeavor. It has been well documented that even if you can bring your conscious mind to direct a particular breathing pattern for a period of time, as soon as your conscious mind focuses elsewhere, or you fall asleep, your breathing reverts naturally to the pattern set by your unconscious mind.

Finally, with our generally heightened consciousness about the dan-gers of radiation exposure, a common concern in respiratory illness is over the risk of radiation involved in a chest X ray. In fact, the radiation exposure from a chest X ray is minimal, much less than the background environmental exposure in many parts of this country. The radiation dose from a single chest X ray is less than one ten-thousandth of a rad (a rad is a unit for measuring radiation), and that is obviously far less than the recommended guidelines for safe yearly radiation exposure (which is one-half a rad). You would need 5,000 chest X rays in one year to reach the recommended guideline for safe exposure to radiation. Even multiple repetitive chest X rays are safe. There have been no documented cases of lung injury or lung cancer from repetitive chest X rays, even in the most seriously ill and closely monitored Intensive Care Unit patients.

TREATMENT CONSIDERATIONS

Because there is no specific treatment to shorten the course of a cold, treatments are symptomatic. Antibiotics kill bacteria, not viruses, and therefore are likely to have no effect on viral colds other than occasionally to upset the stomach. It has been said that the common cold takes one week to resolve naturally and seven days with an antibiotic.

Because the common cold is so common, a great proliferation of over-the-counter cold remedies are available for symptomatic relief, and many are indeed effective. *Antihistamines* exert an antiinflammatory effect and may relieve some nasal congestion. *Decongestants* are medications that constrict the blood vessels, thereby reducing the weeping of fluid from the nasal passages, thus helping to dry a runny nose. Then there are *cough suppressants,* the most effective being codeine and codeine derivatives. Over-the-counter dextromorphan is available in many cold remedies and may be helpful to quiet an irritative cough, particularly at night. Finally, weak topical anesthetics are available in spray and lozenge form to ease the discomfort of a sore throat.

Expectorants are theoretically designed to loosen a cough and promote expectoration of secretions from the respiratory tract. These are generally ineffective and may be sold somewhat ludicrously in combination with a cough suppressant. Generally, secretions that are present in the air tubes will be coughed up by reflex without the aid of any medication.

It is difficult to prevent the spread of viral illnesses through families with small children. Nonetheless, good hygiene at home may be helpful, particularly the practice of covering your mouth when coughing or sneezing, and washing your hands after coming into contact with secretions from the mouth or nose. Viruses are partly spread from one person to the next by little aerosol droplets sprayed into the air, then breathed in by the next victim, and partly from the surface of the hands, which then come in contact with the nose or mouth as a route of entry for the virus.

It has been demonstrated that periods of increased physical and emotional stress are periods of high risk for upper respiratory tract infections within families, and avoiding overexhaustion, either physical or emotional, may in some way protect you from the development of repetitive head colds.

Why some people who smoke heavily escape the ravages of severe emphysema and chronic bronchitis and others do not is unknown. But everyone who smokes is at risk for developing these diseases, and the best prevention is simply not to smoke. Quitting cigarettes is exceedingly difficult for someone addicted to the habit. There is no easy way to break the habit. A number of methods are available, including support groups like Smokenders and other groups sponsored by the American Cancer Society and the American Lung Association. Hypnosis has been effective in some patients, and more recently, Nicorette gum, chewing gum containing nicotine, may be effective when given under medical supervision. What is most important is that you decide to give up smoking and then try any and all methods available. If you fail with one method, try again. Try different techniques—try anything—but do not give up until you actually quit.

The medications used to treat emphysema and chronic bronchitis are much the same as those in asthma. Bronchodilators are given to relieve the contraction of the bronchial muscles that may be narrowing the air tubes, and are effective in relieving shortness of breath. Chest infections may be particularly devastating in people with already serious underlying emphysema and chronic bronchitis, and should be treated immediately with antibiotics. It is particularly important that patients with chronic bronchitis and emphysema receive the pneumococcal vaccine once and a yearly influenza vaccine.

It is often asked whether exercise might injure the lungs or hasten their deterioration. In fact, the answer is no. Sensible exercise can only help to strengthen the heart and the muscles of breathing, as well as contribute to general overall fitness and sense of well-being. It does not in any way injure the lungs even if carried out to the point of huffing and puffing.

In some patients with emphysema and chronic bronchitis, the disease may become so severe that the lungs may become unable to put sufficient amounts of oxygen into the blood; such patients may have persistently low oxygen in the blood despite maximum treatment with bronchodilators. In this case, it has been demonstrated that using oxygen at home will not only improve your capacity to do exercises but can also prolong your life expectancy. To determine if you have persistently low oxygen in the blood, the doctor simply draws a sample of blood from an artery and measures the oxygen content.

FIFTEEN

Muscular/Skeletal Conditions—Risks and Treatment

OSTEOARTHRITIS

Osteoarthritis is the most common rheumatological condition known to man, affecting just about everyone if they are fortunate to live long enough. It is usually described as the disease due to wear and tear. Obviously the longer you live, the more wear and tear your joints get, and the greater the chances you will develop osteoarthritis. Osteoarthritis can also develop after athletic injuries. Joe Namath and Bobby Orr, whose knees are severely damaged from numerous surgeries, have developed osteoarthritis at very early ages.

Another type of osteoarthritis that occurs and that is *not* associated with wear and tear are Heberdens and Bouchard's nodes. These are the lumps that people see near the ends of their fingers. They also appear at the joints in the fingers distal to the knuckles. They begin as painful swellings which eventually evolve to form lumps or nodes, and, after they are formed, the pain resolves but the lumps remain. These are only painful when they form, and are a mild disability that requires no need for any type of surgical repair. They are rarely, if ever, a cause of actual disability, but they can be a source of mild and chronic pain.

Risk Factors

Osteoarthritis nodes run in families. If your mother or grandmother had them, you are at greater risk to develop them. The nodes occur much more commonly in women than in men, but can happen in either sex. However, as is the case with many types of arthritis, women tend to develop this condition more commonly.

Osteoarthritis is a chronic wear-and-tear disorder; as a result, there are no systemic signs. Unlike virtually all the other conditions discussed here, osteoarthritis is restricted to the joints. Thus patients feel none of the symptoms they would if they had rheumatoid arthritis or the other inflammatory conditions.

In osteoarthritis, which is not associated with familial disease, the primary disorder appears to be in the cartilage. The cartilage is the white shiny surface of bone, as is seen on the edge of a chicken bone. Once that cartilage is destroyed by whatever means—be it surgery, age, or wear and tear—it will never grow back. We currently have no medication to make cartilage grow back.

Once the disease starts, the cartilage begins to wear away and the patient begins to feel pain and sometimes swelling. Osteoarthritis is a disease that gets worse with activity, and better with rest. The joints that are usually involved are the more commonly used ones—the knee, hip, the joint at the base of the hand called the first carpometacarpal joint—and, less commonly, the ankle and the shoulder. The elbow joint is almost never involved with osteoarthritis unless there has been prior trauma at this site.

Unless you have had trauma to a joint, or a strong family history of this kind of arthritis, there is no way to predict whether or not you will develop it. As mentioned before, it will occur if you are lucky to live long enough or be very active. How can we prevent you from developing this type of arthritis? Or if you do develop it, how can we prevent it from being quite so severe? There is no way to prevent it; *the only way to forestall any type of arthritis, especially osteoarthritis, is to keep very active, avoid becoming overweight, and keep your muscles in good shape.* This is important in other types of arthritis as well.

Diagnosis

The diagnosis of osteoarthritis can be made clinically, as when a physician looks at your hands and diagnoses Bouchard's nodes without an X ray. Usually, however, the physician will obtain an X ray to make the truly correct diagnosis. At that point he would see the changes caused by osteoarthritis, or any changes that suggest early osteoarthritis, such as loss of cartilage.

Remember that on an X ray you can see only bone and air spaces; you cannot see cartilage. Therefore you can have a damaged cartilage and have a normal X ray. This is important to know, because often the physician will obtain an X ray, tell you it is normal, and then suggest other tests to define whether there are cartilage abnormalities. This is sometimes confusing to patients, as they feel that X rays should unequivocally show whether or not arthritis is present.

Blood tests will not diagnose osteoarthritis, but they may be used to rule out other conditions. The treatment of osteoarthritis depends on the severity. It is one of the many conditions we see in rheumatology where the treatment depends on the degree of pain and/or function loss the patient is experiencing. If the patient has so much pain that he or she cannot sleep at night or cannot walk a few feet (let's say, due to osteoarthritis of the knee), then the doctor may go so far as to suggest total knee replacement or less radical types of surgical procedures. These recommendations are certainly not rare.

In addition to surgery for osteoarthritis, doctors commonly prescribe antiinflammatory medication such as aspirin or some of the higher-priced alternatives—ibuprofen, naproxin, or pyroxicam, to name a few. These may make the pain less or may modify the symptoms, but the medication does not change what will happen once you have this diagnosis. The only thing that *may* change is your ability to keep the joint in good physical shape and keep the muscles surrounding it well-toned. The only other thing that may help slow down the progression of the disease is having the joints do less work: less work meaning less active, traumatizing work, not total absence of exercise. Clearly then, obesity is one of the major things to be changed once the patient does develop osteoarthritis of the knee or hip. Common sense tells us that with less weight to carry, the joint does less work. For each pound that you lose, you decrease the force across the knee by 3 to 4 pounds.

Exercise, weight loss, and continued physical activity are the most beneficial ways to treat osteoarthritis, short of medication or surgery.

Treatment

There is no way that one can prevent osteoarthritis of the hip or knee if you are destined to get it, but by keeping your muscles well-toned, your joints in shape, and maintaining a vigorous exercise program that does not stress the joints, the chances are that your symptoms will be milder. Also, if you do need to have surgery, you will tolerate that more easily and will perform better afterward if you are in good condition.

The best kinds of exercises for people with arthritis are those in which joints are not stressed and there is no more wear and tear than necessary. Obviously, swimming is the ultimate exercise for arthritis. There, not even the weight of gravity is against your joints, and you can move along regularly, toning the muscles as well as improving your cardiovascular fitness. A stationary bicycle or rowing machine is also quite good. Running and court exercises, especially for forestalling knee, ankle, or hip osteoarthritis, are among the worst exercises, although some patients can tolerate the extra stress.

RHEUMATOID ARTHRITIS

The most common type of arthritis that is not due to wear and tear is rheumatoid arthritis. Rheumatoid arthritis is estimated to affect approximately 1 percent of the adult population. In terms of numbers of people, this is a disease that affects over 2 million people in this country alone. The incidence increases with age, and appears to be more common in females by a ratio of almost 2–3 to 1.

This disease is the prototypical inflammatory joint disease, in that the symptoms, which are different than in osteoarthritis, go beyond the joint. It is very important to remember that this is a disease of the *whole* body; the joint only bears the brunt of the majority of the disease. People with rheumatoid arthritis also have systematic manifestations. They feel weak and tired, much like they have the flu. Unfortunately these symptoms do not go away in a week or two.

What separates the joint involvement in this disease from that of osteoarthritis is the presence of morning stiffness. Patients wake up in the morning after a period of restful sleep and take a few hours to feel as good as they are going to feel. They will feel stiff in the morning, have a period of feeling good during the day, and then, commonly, get tired as the day wears on; then they stiffen up again. This is called "gelling," and is a very common manifestation of rheumatoid arthritis. The joints hurt more when they are walked on, but also hurt at rest because there is continued inflammation and swelling in the lining of the joint, or the synovial membrane. Therefore, while osteoarthritis is primarily a disease that begins in the cartilage, rheumatoid arthritis clearly begins in the lining of the joint, the synovium. Only by extension does it then damage bone cartilage, as the inflammatory synovium invades these normal structures.

Diagnosis

The diagnosis of rheumatoid arthritis is a clinical diagnosis, but it is aided by certain laboratory tests; the physician will base the diagnosis mainly on clinical grounds. The patient will have morning stiffness, usually more than three swollen joints, and may have joint fluid or X ray results that are consistent with rheumatoid arthritis. X rays in rheumatoid arthritis will look different from those of osteoarthritis because the disease process begins in a different place.

Laboratory tests are helpful in rheumatoid arthritis. Since it is a disease of the whole body, the patient can be anemic, have a high white blood cell count, or even have mild abnormalities of liver function tests. The sedimentation rate is almost always elevated because there is inflammation involving the entire body.

The test that patients most commonly ask about is the rheumatoid factor. This is not a "truth test." The rheumatoid factor tests one antibody in your blood against another kind of antibody. It is therefore called an "autoantibody." It is important to remember that 85 percent of people with rheumatoid arthritis will have a positive rheumatoid factor, and 15 percent with rheumatoid arthritis who clearly have the disease will not. In addition, 5 to 6 percent of the normal population (and this increases with age) will have a positive test. This is called a false positive. Someone who is 70 years old has an almost 10 percent chance of testing for a positive rhumatoid factor and not having the disease. This is a source of confusion both to physicians and patients, so it is important to remember that the diagnosis is based on both clinical grounds *and* these laboratory tests.

Risk Factors

Rheumatoid arthritis clearly runs in families.It has now been shown that there is clear genetic linkage between a certain type of gene and rheumatoid arthritis. This does not mean that if someone in your family has rheumatoid arthritis you will develop it, but there appears to be one type of rheumatoid arthritis associated with a particular gene profile that can be traced through families. Other risk factors for rheumatoid arthritis include age, in that the incidence appears to increase with age, and sex. Before 60, women tend to get the disease approximately five times more often than men; after age 60 this approaches a 1 to 1 ratio.

Treatment

Once the diagnosis is established, it is quite important for the patient to get effective medical therapy. It has been clearly shown that with good treatment of rheumatoid arthritis, you can change the natural history of the disease and prevent joint damage.

Treatment of rheumatoid arthritis is like building a pyramid. The bottom rung of the pyramid is the use of aspirin or other nonsteroidal agents, as mentioned in the section on osteoarthritis. One builds upon this pyramid, adding medications that are called "slow-acting agents." These may take months to work, but if they do they will slow down the progression of rheumatoid arthritis. These medications include: hydroxychloroquine, which is an antimalarial, gold salt therapy, an injection or pill that is quite effective for rheumatoid arthritis, or penicillamine tablets. These latter groups of medicines all have side effects (adverse reactions), some of which can be very serious. "Newer" agents include methetrexate and azathioprine.

Corticosteroids, or steroids, are used quite commonly and are quite beneficial in some patients. However, they have numerous side effects including cataracts, hair growth, obesity, hypertension, diabetes, and susceptibility to infection and osteoporosis. Still, with judicious use—hopefully on an every-other-morning schedule—they are very useful as an adjunct to the above-mentioned agents. The physician and the patient should always be trying to use the minimum dose when it's necessary to use steroids at all.

There is a $2 to $3 billion quackery industry in the treatment of arthritis, and most of these "medicines" are used for the treatment of rheumatoid arthritis or osteoarthritis. These can be as simple as hanging garlic from your neck, wearing copper bracelets, taking bee venom, castor oil, cocaine, and other types of exotic therapies, and diets. Diet has never been shown to change the natural history of rheumatoid arthritis or osteoarthritis, nor have any of these other therapies. Vitamins have never been shown to change the natural history of the disease either. Patients do feel compelled to try some of these alternate agents or therapies, which include fad diets and mega-vitamins, but it is important to tell your physician about any alternative therapy that you choose, because some can be very harmful from a medical standpoint.

There is no way that you can keep yourself from developing rheumatoid arthritis, but certainly the measures mentioned regarding osteoarthritis—to keep in shape and keep your muscles well-toned—are quite essential. Rheumatoid arthritis is an illness in which self-help groups and organizations are often quite useful. Patients do need to talk to other patients about a chronic disease such as rheumatoid arthritis. The best source of help with this condition (and virtually all other conditions mentioned in this chapter) is the Arthritis Foundation; it has chapters throughout the entire country and is a good resource for patients. Literature on arthritis is given out by the foundation at little cost or for free. The main address of the Arthritis Foundation is: 1314 Spring Street N.W., Atlanta, Ga. 30309.

LUPUS

Risk Factors

Systematic lupus erythematosus (SLE or lupus) is a protean disease with diffuse symptoms that are seemingly unrelated, numerous, and can occur over many years' time. The disease is also fairly common, being approximately one-tenth as common as rheumatoid arthritis. It also tends to affect females more than males by a ratio of 5 to 1. Lupus is more common and more severe in black patients and black females, with the ratio of black-to-white incidence at 4 to 1. Lupus tends to occur in young women, ages 20 to 40, and when it does occur in older patients it tends to be relatively more benign.

Lupus also runs in families and, like rheumatoid arthritis, is associated with its own particular genetic marker. But again, as in rheumatoid arthritis, this is not definitive. Some families will have a high incidence of lupus, but in others there will be only sporadic cases.

Diagnosis

The American Rheumatism Association has a classification for lupus in which the diagnosis is based on numerous laboratory tests as well as the following symptoms (the more signs present, the more likely the disease is present):

- rash along the face in a "butterfly pattern," under the eyes and over the bridge of the nose
- rash with scarring on the face or other parts of the sun-exposed skin
- photosensitivity to the extent that the patient gets ill on sun exposure
- ulcers in the mouth
- arthritis involving two or more joints
- "serositis" or inflammation in the stomach
- chest pain on deep breathing or on coughing
- kidney disease
- neurologic abnormalities such as seizures and various laboratory abnormalities including low white blood cell count, low platelet count, anemia, or positive lab tests called the ANA, or antinuclear antibodies.

The definitive lab test for lupus is the ANA. If this lab test is positive, the patient has a circulating antibody against the nucleus of human cells and other cells. Ninety-nine percent of all patients with SLE have this antibody, but again, as in rheumatoid arthritis, there are many normal patients (5 percent) who have a positive test but do not have the disease.

Patients with lupus often will have numerous symptoms as mentioned above which can be present for a number of months to years before the diagnosis is made. Patients will have fever, fatigue, or ulcers, possible illness on sun exposure, and rashes, and see many doctors before the diagnosis of SLE is made. The arthritis in lupus tends to be relatively mild but it can be very annoying. The disease can affect the kidneys and can progress to kidney failure, but there is evidence that with aggressive followup and treatment with corticosteroids or, rarely, immunosuppressive agents, this can be forestalled.

Treatment

The only current treatment for lupus is to treat the symptoms as they develop. Patients with lupus should almost always use sunscreens with protection value of at least "15" if it can be obtained. The skin rash is treated with topical corticosteroids, and the arthritis and skin are both treated with the same agent used in rheumatoid arthritis, hydroxychloroquine. In addition, nonsteroidal antiinflammatory agents or aspirin are quite useful for the muscle pain as well as the arthritis of SLE.

If severe systemic symptoms develop, such as kidney disease or neurological disease, or even if fever and lethargy become a problematic symptom, various doses of corticosteroids can be used. There are inherent problems with the use of these agents, but with this disease, even more so than with others discussed earlier, the treatment can be life-saving. These are the only treatments that are efficacious; again, home remedies as mentioned in the discussion on rheumatoid arthritis can be useful for the patient but can in no way help medically.

The lupus patient needs to get rest, as fatigue is a very prominent part of the illness. Afternoon naps, if possible, or at least rest periods, are certainly useful. It is also important for the young female patient to realize that pregnancy in patients with lupus does have certain risks: There is an increased risk of fetal mortality and there is a risk that the mother may have a difficult time in the third trimester and the postpartum period, particularly with worsening of kidney and neurologic disease. However, with appropriate medical management one can carry a child to term and have a successful outcome.

The Lupus and Arthritis foundations are both prime examples of resources for patients. They distribute literature and organize self-help groups.

GOUT

Risk Factors

One of the more common diseases that our population encounters is gout. Gout is the name for that type of arthritis caused by deposition of uric acid crystals in the synovium, or lining of the joints, which then causes inflammation in that particular joint. The lab test for gout is an elevated uric acid. There is a very complex interplay of multiple factors in the development of gout, including sex, age, and diet. This type of arthritis is different from others in that diet can play a role. Anything that will raise your uric acid level can increase your likelihood of getting gout; some of the factors that raise uric acid are foods that are high in protein—liver and beef—and alcohol, which inhibits your kidneys' ability to excrete uric acid. When uric acid gets above a certain level, approximately 10 mg percent in the blood, there is a higher probability of developing a gout attack than at lower levels.

Other factors that contribute to gout are the patient's sex and endocrine status. It has been noted for many years, as far back as Hippocrates' time, that women do not usually develop gout until after menopause, and that males do not develop gout until after puberty. This has certainly held true. Additional factors that are related to the development of gout in our society are the use of drugs such as thiazide diuretics, which raise uric acid.

Treatment

The treatment of an acute gout attack involves antiinflammatory drugs, draining fluid from the joints, or simple watchful waiting, as most gout attacks do resolve themselves in seven to fourteen days. There is preventive treatment for chronic gout with a medication called alopurinol, which decreases production of uric acid, and there is also a medication called probenecid, which increases excretion of uric acid through the kidneys. Diet certainly can play a role, but with these medications it is not usually necessary in this day and age to have patients avoid any particular foods. However, it may be possible to decrease gout attacks by zealous dietary measures; dietary treatments may be helpful in patients who cannot take the medications. In addition, daily treatment with colchicine decreased gout attacks without changing uric acid flux.

Diagnosis of gout is not made by an elevated serum uric acid, but is made by observing repetitive joint attacks that are painful, involve swelling, and which resolve without any joint destruction. Diagnosis can also be made by the demonstration of uric acid crystals in the joint. A high serum uric acid is suggestive of gout but not diagnostic proof.

POLYMYALGIA RHEUMATICA

A common condition that we are now seeing more and more frequently, especially in the population over 60, is polymyalgia rheumatica. This syndrome is defined as the onset, usually suddenly or within one month, of acute pain or stiffness in the approximal shoulder or hip girdle. The patient will have profound fatigue and weakness, and this disease may be associated with an inflammatory disease of the arteries called "giant cell arteritis." If that is the case, the patient will have severe headaches, diseases of the great vessels in the chest and heart, and, rarely, blindness. Occasionally there may be a bland and mild arthritis. This disease is diagnosed with the help of physician awareness and the observation of a marked elevation of the sedimentation rate blood test.

With this pattern of illness present and with an elevated sedimentation rate, the physician can treat this disease quite successfully with low doses of corticosteroids. Doses of prednisone 10 to 15 mg daily are usually adequate to suppress the symptoms totally and with time (occasionally many years) the patient can be treated successfully. Occasionally medication can be stopped. This disease must be considered in elderly patients with the disease pattern mentioned above, as there can be a prolonged course of disability and pain before the diagnosis is made. The disease can occasionally be treated with some of the nonsteroidal antiinflammatory medicines already mentioned. However, if the diagnosis of giant cell arteries is entertained, one should consider judicious use of corticosteroids, because of a risk of blindness.

BACK PAIN: STRUCTURAL AND INFLAMMATORY

Diagnosis

Back pain is the price that we must pay for walking upright. This places a rather undue stress on our musculature and with time causes weakening of ligamentous attachments and, eventually, in some people, a disk herniation. In addition, there is a large group of illnesses not related to the mechanical stress which can cause back pain. These are inflammatory disorders that start from the sacroiliac joint and march all the way up to the neck.

Low Back Pain

The most common problem that people have is simple low back strain; at its worst this is called sciatica. It is very common for patients to get the terms "sciatica" and "disk herniation" confused, but basically the pathophysiology is the same for the two. There is a weakening in the back, or arthritis forms in its joints, and either a disk that separates vertebrae protrudes and pinches the sciatic nerve, or there is extra bony growth around these joints which over time builds up and protrudes upon the nerve. When the nerve is stimulated, the pain proceeds down the affected extremity. Increased use causes this pain to become worse, and rest tends to make it better. Low back pain that spreads to the buttocks is properly called sciatica.

Low back pain is the prototypical disorder that can be modulated. Active exercise, specifically those exercises strengthening the lower back and abdominal muscles, may be able to prevent or forestall problems with your lower back. The abdominal muscles, when they are strengthened, supply extra support for your paravertebral or back muscles, and in this way can take some of the "stress" off the disk and back and help prevent further back damage. For purely mechanical back pain, other measures that can be taken include appropriate physical conditioning, avoidance of bending and stooping, and learning to lift things with the legs instead of the back.

Treatment

Once a diagnosis of acute low back pain, sciatica, or disk disease is made, the appropriate treatment is absolute bed rest. There are no magic tricks—patients and physicians should be aware of that. The sudden onset of sciatica does not mean the patient needs to have back surgery, but to get appropriate relief the patient should basically go to bed for seven to ten days, take effective analgesics such as aspirin or stronger medication, possibly use muscle relaxants, and simply give it time before any panic buttons are pushed.

When a person with lower back pain first sees a physician, X rays are not indicated at all unless the pain is not relieved in a short period of time, the patient is older, or the patient has other medical problems. Standard types of back pain do not run in families, and do cut across all categories of Western men and women, regardless of ethnic background. Age is a prime consideration because with time, as in osteoarthritis, we develop arthritis in our lumbosacral spine as well as disk degeneration, and we can then develop disk herniation or chronic back problems.

As mentioned before, with back diseases, staying in proper physical shape with continued exercise for abdominal and lower back muscles can forestall this from becoming a chronic problem. If pain continues despite adequate therapy, or if neurological changes or bladder or bowel problems develop, one must consider surgery. Unless there are neurological problems or bladder or bowel problems, the decision to have surgery is up to the patient—it is a "quality of life" decision. If you undergo surgery for relief of pain, you should be cognizant of the fact that 80 percent of such surgery is successful and 20 percent is not. In addition, you should be aware that there are obvious complications of back surgery and general anesthesia, and once those risks are considered, surgery can be safely performed.★

The patient must be aware of these risks, because some patients prefer to live with the chronic pain rather than have surgery. Other treatment modalities that are not "conventional" that have been used for back pain include transcutaneous nerve stimulators, which are useful as pain therapy adjuncts; corsets, which are also quite useful to support the back; acupuncture; and epideral steroid injections. This latter group of treatment can be quite useful and occasionally can postpone or prevent surgery.

OTHER BACK PAIN

Other causes of back pain, which are not mechanical or diskogeneic and which should absolutely not be treated surgically, are the group of spondylitis. This group is a wide variety of illnesses including ankylosing spondylitis, Reiter's, and other back conditions associated with inflammatory bowel disease or other rheumatic disease. The most common of these is ankylosing spondylitis (A.S.). It tends more often than not to be a disease of young men, but women can be affected as well.

Risk Factors for A.S.

One definitely inherits a predisposition for A.S. There is a gene that is passed on from generation to generation which, upon encountering something "in our environment" (be it an infection or an environmental influence), sets up a series of reactions resulting in low back pain. What characterizes the low back pain of spondylitis versus the low back pain of diskogenic disease is the youthful age of the patient,

---

★ Diagnostic tests such as the CAT scan and myelogram aid the surgeon in selecting appropriate candidates for an operation. You should satisfy yourself that the surgeon you have selected has answered all your questions and has a good reputation. Both orthopedists and neurosurgeons do back surgery.

morning stiffness, and improvement with use. People with disk-type diseases may get worse with use and better with rest, whereas the patient with an inflammatory back condition such as spondylitis will improve with use and get worse after prolonged periods of inactivity.

Treatment

Treatment for A.S., again, is related to very active physical therapy, strengthening "antigravity muscles" in and around the back, avoidance of inappropriate posture, and judicious use of corsets, bedboards, and so on. A.S. and the other diseases causing spondylitis, as in rheumatoid arthritis, is a systematic disease, and as a result can effect the patient's feeling of well-being, resulting in fatigue and weight loss. In addition, although rarely, patients can have bowel symptoms, urinary tract symptoms, or even ocular symptoms.

There is no cure for this particular illness, but with nonsteroidal antiinflammatory agents, active use of physical therapy, and continuing physical activity, patients almost always do well. To differentiate between the various back conditions, the physician will make a diagnosis on the basis of the clinical evidence, considering the differences outlined above. In addition, X rays can be very useful in diagnosis. The X ray for A.S. or other types of inflammatory back conditions would look totally different from the X ray for common problems of disk disease in the back, or for other conditions resembling osteoarthritis in the spine. This is one instance in which X rays can give a definitive answer.

OSTEOPOROSIS

One of the more common disorders that should be discussed is a disorder that affects virtually every woman in this country—osteoporosis. Osteoporosis means thin bones; the body is not putting enough protein into the bone to calcify them. Numerous factors are associated with osteoporosis, but the most common appears to be lack of estrogen. Other factors that always have to be investigated when someone makes a diagnosis of osteoporosis are the amount of calcium intake, sun exposure, vitamin D intake, or the presence of concomitant illnesses. These can give the physician an idea that the diagnosis is not osteoporosis, but may in fact be another similar bone disease, called "osteomalacia."

Osteomalacia is the result of a lack of mineralization, not a lack of protein. It has now been well demonstrated that women after menopause and men (at a much slower rate) after age 30 to 35 begin to lose bone mass. It is this prolonged loss of bone mass over time that would cause osteoporosis, weak bones, and the eventual compression fractures and occasional deformities that we see in our elder population.

The most important thing about osteoporosis is that much of it can be avoided. There are medical as well as physical therapies that may forestall the development of this dreaded complication of age. The average bone mass is greater in black women than in white women or women of Asian descent; therefore, white women and Oriental-Asian women are at higher risk for development of osteoporosis. It also does appear that there is an increased familial risk, but this is hard to separate from the facts above.

Once a woman does approach menopause, there are ways that she may be able to forestall the development of osteoporosis. It has now been found that exercise is one of the main stimuli to make more bone mass. If someone simply lies in bed or does not use an extremity, his or her bones will slowly decalcify and the result will be osteoporosis, weak bones, and eventual fractures. Therefore, appropriate exercise is probably as important if not more important than any medications to forestall the development of osteoporosis. Simple walking exercises for prolonged periods three to four times a week are enough. Patients do not need to be jogging or doing extraordinarily strenuous physical exercise. *Simple* exercise cannot be overdone and its importance cannot be overestimated.

Estrogen treatment should also be used judiciously. Women with premature surgical menopause—removal of ovaries surgically—should all be uniformly treated with appropriate estrogens and/or progesterones. There is some evidence that use of the hormone may result in an increased risk of endometrial cancer or thrombophlebitis, and even though this risk may be small, it is deemed necessary to prevent the possibly greater problem of osteoporosis.

Calcium intake should also be maintained. Patients should take a minimum dose of 1000–1500 mg of calcium per day. Calcium preparations are now available over the counter and include oyster shell calcium, calcium tartrate or lactate, or even Tums (calcium carbonate). Five Tums tablets a day would supply 1000 mg of calcium. The best way to maximize calcium intake, however, is dietary. Four glasses—at least a quart—of milk a day would be enough to maintain the adequate calcium and vitamin D that is necessary for most patients. Low-fat or skim milk should be used to avoid calories and fat.

Large doses of vitamin D are not necessary, and most patients with osteoporosis would just be wise to make sure they are getting appropriate vitamin D, either through dietary measures or simply by taking a standard multivitamin which has the 100 percent MDR for vitamin D.

Other measures that are possibly useful in the treatment of osteoporosis include fluoride, but this is still relatively experimental, and so far the appropriate fluoride tablets have not been marketed for use. Calcitonin, a human hormone, is also occasionally used.

Diagnosis

The diagnosis of osteoporosis is not an easy one. The physician takes an X ray of the affected bone, usually in the back, and sees "thin bones." The radiologist calls this "osteopenia," or thin bones. The physician must then decide, with the help of a series of lab tests of the blood as well as occasional urine tests, whether this osteopenia is osteoporosis or osteomalacia. In rare cases, the physician may even have to do a bone biopsy to define precisely whether the primary problem is osteoporosis or osteomalacia. Usually this is not necessary, and with simple X rays, some blood studies, and sometimes urine studies the physician can make the correct diagnosis of osteoporosis or osteomalacia. Dual photon densitometry and quantitative CT scans can diagnose osteoporosis earlier than standard X rays.

In summary, adequate hormonal replacement, calcium, vitamin D, and, most important, continued physical exercise may forestall or prevent much of the osteoporosis that we see in our population.

OTHER CONDITIONS

There are numerous other muscular/skeletal conditions that afflict our population, including tendinitis and bursitis. The most common locations to have tendinitis or bursitis are in the shoulder, elbow, hip, or knee area. There are various tendons and bursa that can become painful and swollen for reasons that are not entirely clear. Usually these are related to normal wear and tear; the injury somehow creates an inflammatory process and pain. Some of the more common types of bursitis or tendinitis are tennis elbow; trochanteric bursitis, or a pain of the hip area, and housemaid's knee.

These illnesses are all diagnosed by a physical exam. X rays are rarely necessary, though they may be obtained to confirm that the underlying joint is not involved. Treatment includes, again, the use of aspirin or nonsteroidal antiinflammatory drugs, or local modalities; steroids pills or injections are rarely used. R.I.C.E.—Rest, Ice, and Elevation—is commonly used; the rule of thumb regarding these modalities is that after an acute injury the patient should use R.I.C.E. for 48 hours, but not for any prolonged period of time. The importance of physical therapy, specifically for shoulder disorders, cannot be overemphasized. Appropriate and aggressive physical therapy will continue to improve the motion in one's shoulder despite bursitis and tendinitis.

Other forms of arthritis that doctors commonly see can be quite severe and life-threatening. These include diseases such as progressive systemic sclerosis or scleroderma, which is associated with a relatively common abnormality called Reynaud's phenomenon. This is where the extremities change color when exposed to cold—first they become white, then bluish, then red. More often than not this is a benign syndrome occurring in young females, which is more of a nuisance than a problem. However, it may be a prodrome or warning sign of the development of scleroderma. This can affect the skin with tightening and can eventually affect internal organs, including the kidneys, as well as the lungs and the heart. Polymyositis and dermatomyositis are rare conditions that cause inflammation of the muscles, profound weakness, and pain and swelling. Systemic symptoms, once again, can be prominent in both of these illnesses—fatigue, weakness, and malaise, as well as arthritis. Diagnosis of scleroderma is made on clinical grounds but the diagnosis of polymyositis is made by blood studies, muscle tests, and possibly muscle biopsies. Treatment of both of these conditions includes treating the resultant problem (for example, hypertension) and using corticosteroids for treatment of polymyositis. The Arthritis Foundation, once again, is a prime resource for the patient with any of these illnesses, and there are scleroderma support groups which can be organized and/or discovered through this organization.

The rheumatic diseases encompass virtually every segment of our population, and arthritis is a very common problem, affecting millions of people in our society. Only with appropriate early diagnosis, judicious use of medication and physical therapy, and patient education can some of the disabling aspects of these conditions be forestalled and lessened. An appropriate resource for information on all of these measures is your local Arthritis Foundation.

Common Gastrointestinal Disorders

Here are some of the more common G.I. disorders, which can be treated or prevented.

REFLUX ESOPHAGITIS

This is often associated with belching an acid taste into the mouth, nausea, stomach discomfort, or a burning sensation usually within one hour of eating. It often occurs when lying down or when stooping or lifting. People with hiatus hernia often have reflux esophagitis.

HERPETIC ESOPHAGITIS

Symptoms are pain on swallowing or vomiting blood, often related to oral herpes due to sexual transmission.

CHRONIC GASTRITIS

This condition occurs more frequently as we age. It may be present with anemia or be entirely asymptomatic until complicated with gastric cancer. There is a higher incidence of the disease among certain families, especially those of northern European background. Susceptibility to cancer may be related to nitrites and nitrous compounds, such as those in bacon and spinach, or combinations of these in the diet.

PANCREATITIS

First signs occur with the development of a sudden severe abdominal pain above the navel, which travels through to the back. Accompanying symptoms may include a low-grade temperature, nausea, and vomiting. People at risk are men, consumers of excessive amounts of alcohol, those with gallstone disease (not always known), or those on medications that may in rare cases cause pancreatitis.

GASTRIC CANCER

This form of cancer is more common in males than females, with a higher incidence occurring in northern industrial areas. Studies have shown changes in incidence related to migration from high- to low-risk areas, and vice versa; this suggests environmental factors. There is also an association with starch, pickled vegetables, salted fish, and meats containing nitrates and nitrous compounds. Furthermore there is a relationship to people with blood group A, over age 50, and from black and lower socioeconomic groups. The risk is reduced by a diet using whole milk, fresh vegetables, and vitamin C.

GASTRIC ULCERS

Peak incidence occurs in those between 55 and 65 years of age. Symptoms consist of poorly localized pain below the rib cage, usually within three hours of eating. Gastric ulcer pain can be relieved by food or by antacids. Some weight loss is common among ulcer patients. Related to aspirin ingestion, possibly acetaminophen, and smoking cigarettes. There are conflicting theories regarding the effects of stress from life's events. There is a threefold increased risk of incidence in relatives of gastric ulcer patients.

IRRITABLE BOWEL SYNDROME

This condition occurs more frequently in females, Caucasians, and Jews under age 35. The symptoms are divided between abdominal pain with constipation and diarrhea. Often constipation may alternate with diarrhea, although sometimes the patient may have painless diarrhea only. Symptoms often begin in late adolescence. The associated constipation eventually leads to increasing use of laxatives and even enemas. The patient's stools generally are hard, narrow, and fragmented, causing pain that usually increases with duration and severity of constipation. Often there is a history of incomplete relief from evacuation. Patients often may have a normal bowel movement followed by increasingly loose stools. Variable pain may be partially relieved by bowel movements. The dull and aching but frequently cramping and sharp pain is often precipitated by meals. Accompanying symptoms include bloating, belching, and vomiting and an inability to eat large meals. I.B.S. is often—though not always—related to stress, anxiety, or depression.

SEXUALLY TRANSMITTED DISEASES

These are an unfortunate consequence of the sexual revolution and new attitudes regarding sexual practices. These diseases may involve not only the genitalia but also the digestive tract, particularly the rectum. Many intestinal infections may be transmitted by sexual contact. While some may have serious consequences, the majority do not. Shigellosis, giardiasis, and amebiasis are the most commonly transmitted through sexual contact. In this situation a person may transmit the disease after inadequate washing of hands. Food or water then becomes contaminated, resulting in infection to the contacted person.

Symptoms of these sexual infections generally include watery or even bloody diarrhea associated with severe abdominal pain. Symptoms may last from days to weeks without treatment. Gonorrhea or herpes or other sexual diseases can only be transmitted by direct sexual contact. Herpes may produce sores and pain around the anus and rectum. As these are sexually transmitted diseases of sexually active individuals, they predominantly affect people between the ages 20 and 50. They are more likely to occur as a result of casual sexual liaisons.

INFLAMMATORY BOWEL DISEASE

This refers to ulcerative colitis, proctitis, and Crohn's disease. They have no known etiologies, although viruses and altered immunity are currently being investigated. Ulcerative colitis is an inflammation of the colon. In its more limited form, confined to the rectum, it is referred to as ulcerative proctitis. The diarrhea involved is different from the usual type; it is generally bloody and chronic. It is often associated with weight loss and loss of appetite.

ULCERATIVE COLITIS

This disease has two peak periods, one in adolescence and one in the fifth decade of life. There is a higher incidence among Jews than non-Jews and a lower incidence among blacks than whites. Family incidence is also higher.

CROHN'S DISEASE

This inflammatory disorder, sometimes known as ileitis may involve the small and/or large intestine. Unlike ulcerative colitis, Crohn's diarrhea usually occurs without the presence of blood. Weight loss, anorexia, and abdominal pain are associated symptoms. It, too, is more common in Jews and there is a higher familial incidence. The most frequent age at onset is between 15 and 30.

DIVERTICULOSIS

A condition present in as many as 50 percent of the population at age 60, diverticulosis, when it does produce symptoms, commonly produces alternating constipation and diarrhea. Generally, however, it is silent until inflammation or bleeding occurs. If one of the diverticula, or pouches along the intestinal wall, becomes infected or inflamed, then severe pain may result, accompanied by fever, nausea, and vomiting.

Occasionally small blood vessels at the base of a pouch become disrupted, and there may be significant gastrointestinal bleeding. Diverticulosis is a condition peculiar to Western civilization, with its diets that are low in fiber and high in refined foods. It is well known that African populations, which consume diets high in crude fiber, rarely develop diverticulosis. There also may be a higher incidence of diverticulosis in those with irritable bowel syndrome.

INTESTINAL POLYPS

These abnormal growths of tissue may occur anywhere in the G.I. tract but are usually in the large intestine. Symptoms of polyps generally occur after they've developed, producing variable amounts of bleeding, most of which is not even visible to the naked eye. Polyps are rare in underdeveloped countries, suggesting that our low-fiber diets are partially responsible for their presence. They are also found more frequently in those individuals whose families have a higher incidence of polyps and cancer of the colon.

COLON CANCER

In its earliest stages colon cancer is silent. Only when the cancer enlarges will the symptoms become evident; it may produce bleeding, invisible to the naked eye, which can result in anemia. Its other predominant symptom is a change in bowel habits, often accompanied by abdominal pain, weakness, anorexia, and weight loss. The risk for colon cancer increases with age, doubling with each decade after 40 years. People at high risk are those with a family history of colon cancer, a history of polyps, female genital cancer, or ulcerative colitis.

HEMORRHOIDS

Hemorrhoids are the most common cause of rectal bleeding, although any abnormality of the gastrointestinal tract may cause it. Hemorrhoids are actually dilated veins of the passageway of the lower rectum and anus; 50 percent of the population over 50 has hemorrhoids. Populations at risk for hemorrhoids are those with diets low in fiber. Straining at defecation to evacuate hard stools also seems to promote their development. Most people with mildly symptomatic hemorrhoids will do better with a high-residue diet, and defecation that is as prompt as possible with little strain.

CONSTIPATION

This name is given to infrequent or difficult evacuation of small hard stools. It is a common condition that predominantly affects the very young and the aged. While the number of bowel movements is variable in the general population, a normal individual should pass at least three stools per week. Constipation is important and should be recognized because of the enormous economic and social costs. Interestingly, in the not too distant past people underwent enemas at regular intervals in spas or even removal of the colon for constipation. Sufferers will often not have complaints of constipation but rather abdominal discomfort, stomach rumbling, loss of appetite, nausea, and malaise.

HEPATITIS

While jaundice is the best-known hallmark of this disease, only 10 percent of all patients with hepatitis will develop it. In fact, the condition may be completely without symptoms. However, symptoms such as skin rash, loss of appetite, muscle and joint aches, nausea, vomiting, low-grade fever, and darkening of the urine are often important warning signs.

Hepatitis may be transmitted by any of several viruses, and depending on the virus, it may be passed within families or by sexual contacts. Inadequate washing of hands after exposure to an individual who carries the disease, contact with contaminated food or water, and blood transfusions are the most common means of contracting hepatitis.

CIRRHOSIS

Cirrhosis may not cause any symptoms whatsoever. While alcohol is commonly implicated as the chief culprit, cirrhosis may also occur in a small percentage of patients exposed to a variety of substances, including certain drugs; to those virsues that cause hepatitis; and for certain reasons that are still unclear. Symptoms that do appear with cirrhosis may include bleeding from varicose veins of the esophagus. Other symptoms might include a change of mental status, with irritability, alteration of the sleep-wake cycle, or development of a distended abdomen due to fluid retention. Liver cancer can infrequently complicate cirrhosis of the liver.

HOW WE KNOW WHAT'S WRONG— DIAGNOSIS AND G.I. TESTS

Several tests are commonly used to diagnose stomach and digestive disorders. These are often referred to as G.I. (gastrointestinal) tests, and can be divided into blood tests, stool analyses, X-ray procedures, and fiberoptic instrumentation tests.

All G.I. procedures can be performed in a hospital outpatient department or in your doctor's office. The patient should always ask the physician about diagnosis and whether certain tests are really necessary.

For example, an ulcer can be diagnosed either by X-ray procedures, which are the most cost-effective, or by fiberoptic instrumentation, which generally requires sedation and the loss of at least one day's work.

Generally speaking, G.I. therapy should never be instituted without a specific diagnosis from your doctor. For every case of abdominal discomfort related to ulcer disease, there are ten cases for which the discomfort is simply related to diet or stress alone. Treating the patient with an antiulcer drug only on the basis of symptoms and without adequate diagnostic testing could lead to unnecessary drug reactions or other unpleasant side effects.

In general, G.I. tests are performed to *rule out* a G.I. illness. The following are the most common:

Barium Swallow or Upper G.I. Series: Performed to rule out the presence of an inflammation of the esophagus or stomach, or the presence of an ulcer in the stomach and duodenum. A white chalky substance is swallowed by the patient. Its passage through the esophagus, stomach, and intestine is checked by an X-ray test, so the total radiation involved can be substantial. Approximately 80 to 90 percent of all ulcers are diagnosed in this fashion.

Barium Enema or Lower G.I Series: A chalky substance (such as barium) is inserted rectally in an enema to evaluate the large intestine for causes of diarrhea, rectal bleeding, or abdominal pain. As many patients have difficulty retaining the barium, a balloon attached to the enema tubing is inflated to prevent defecation.

Upper Endoscopy: A flexible fiberoptic tube called an endoscope is passed through the mouth to observe the esophagus, stomach, and duodenum directly. These instruments contain channels through which instruments can be easily inserted without pain for the patient. Biopsies—snippets of tissue—may be taken at the same time if abnormal areas are seen. This procedure is frequently used when upper G.I. test results suggest an abnormality of the esophagus or stomach, or when a patient is bleeding in the upper intestinal area.

Sigmoidoscopy or Colonoscopy: A rigid tube called a sigmoidoscope is passed through the rectum into one side of the colon. The colonoscope is a flexible fiberoptic tube that can pass through the entire colon. These procedures are generally used in combination with the barium enema, either in a preventive fashion to check for polyps or cancer or to take biopsies when the patient has a puzzling form of diarrhea or rectal bleeding.

Abdominal Ultrasound: Test soundwaves are transmitted from an ultrasound machine on the surface of the abdomen to evaluate internal organs, such as the gallbladder, liver, pancreas, uterus, and ovaries.

The CAT Scan: This is a more sophisticated X-ray procedure to observe the internal organs. It should be used with caution on patients allergic to iodine or IVP dye, which is injected to trace the picture on the X ray.

TREATMENT

Reflux Esophagitis: Therapy is divided into short- and long-term approaches. When heartburn develops, liquid antacids are effective in relieving the discomfort. Should none be available, water is an acceptable alternative. Almost anything that increases pressure in the abdomen may result in heartburn. Therefore, symptoms can be controlled by weight loss in the overweight individual and avoidance of tight clothing and bending over; elevation of the head of the bed by 30 degrees is also effective. Eating smaller amounts of food more often can also decrease symptoms, as well as avoiding lying down until two to three hours after eating. Additionally, certain foods may increase heartburn, such as chocolate, coffee, tea, citrus fruits, alcohol, and those that are high in fat. Smoking should also be avoided.

Herpetic Esophagitis: Treated with topical anesthetics and clear liquids. More recently a new medication (Acyclovar) may decrease the duration of an initial attack.

Chronic Gastritis: There is no known therapy for this ailment.

Pancreatitis: During an acute attack the patient is hospitalized and given intravenous feedings only; the pain is treated with analgesics. If the symptoms are caused by gallstone disease, then the gallbladder should be removed. If alcohol is responsible, its use should be stopped completely and immediately. Any drugs responsible should be avoided.

Gastric Ulcer: Therapy is directed toward a reduction of acid produced by the stomach. Antacids can buffer the acid produced, and other medications, such as Tagamet (cimetidine), decrease the amount of acid produced. In the near future so-called "protective" drugs will be marketed that can heal ulcers and prevent their recurrence; these work by protecting the lining of the stomach from acid. Whatever form of therapy is employed, however, close followup by either upper endoscopy or X rays is required, since gastric cancer can occasionally resemble the benign gastric ulcer. Nonhealing of gastric ulcers after two to three months may indicate that surgery is needed.

Gastric Cancer: Surgery is currently the only effective form of therapy.

Duodenal Ulcer: As with gastric ulcers, current therapy is directed toward reducing stomach acid. Smoking and alcohol should be avoided. It was previously felt that food was an important part of ulcer treatment; however, extensive studies have shown that bland diets or milk do not improve healing rates. Specific foods that cause an increase in discomfort in the individual are those to be avoided.

Irritable Bowel Syndrome: Treatment includes an appropriate diet with adequate exercise. Medication is used only as a final measure. Since irritable bowel syndrome generally results from diets that are low in fiber and high in fat, dietary changes should be made that ensure high fiber (foods such as whole wheat, bran, fiber supplements, vegetables) and low fat content. Often, though, diets that are high in vegetable fiber (the cabbage family, particularly) may exacerbate the symptoms by producing gas and distention. For those individuals affected, these foods should be avoided. Much has been made of the contribution of stress to irritable bowel syndrome. These concerns would appear to be legitimate, and stress-reducing measures may be helpful.

Sexually Transmitted Disease: The therapy depends on the given infection. When these diseases are suspected a physician should be consulted immediately.

Inflammatory Bowel Diseases: These are generally chronic diseases without known cures. Presently, therapy is directed toward control of symptoms. When there are acute flareups, avoidance of stimulants such as caffeine, citrus fruits, and high roughage is recommended. Current medical therapy includes steroids and Azulfidine (sulfasalazine), which control symptoms and often produce long-term remissions. Steroids should be used only when necessary, under a physician's guidance, to avoid serious side effects such as high blood pressure, diabetes, weakening of bone architecture, and infections. Antidiarrheal medications such as Kaopectate, Lomotil, and Imodium should be used with caution.

Diverticulosis: Diets high in fiber content are effective in reducing symptoms and decreasing further progression of the disease.

Intestinal Polyps: No current therapy is known to prevent recurrence. Fat content in the diet should be reduced by 25 percent, and fiber-containing foods should be consumed on a daily basis. Followup is essential, so if polyps are present they can be removed on an outpatient basis via the fiberoptic instruments mentioned earlier.

Colon Cancer: Surgery is the only effective treatment.

Hepatitis: Although there is no known therapy, people at high risk for developing hepatitis, such as laboratory workers, workers in institutions for the mentally retarded, and spouses of patients with hepatitis, should be treated with gamma globulin and/or vaccines.

Cirrhosis: Treated by avoiding alcohol and other sedatives that are detoxified by the liver.

Hemorrhoids: Most people with mildly symptomatic hemorrhoids will respond to a high-residue diet, defecating as promptly as possible with as little strain as possible. Ointments and rectal suppositories are of limited value. In people who have more severe symptoms, rubber-band ligation, cryosurgery, or injection therapy should be attempted prior to surgical removal.

Constipation: Treatment is fairly simple and can be readily initiated by the patients themselves:

First, it is essential to stop taking laxatives and enemas. A diet high in fiber with at least 14 grams of crude fiber per day, as well as adequate exercise and regular use of the toilet, is important. Should these measures fail to work, then consultation with a physician is necessary to rule out organic causes of constipation, such as drugs, diabetes, hypothyroidism, or colon problems.

ALTERNATIVE THERAPIES

Alternative forms of management include dietary, manipulative, Oriental, or psychological therapies.

Naturopaths believe that by following their general guidelines, the digestive system can realign itself and the symptoms will disappear. For example, hemorrhoids are related to secondary constipation; this is corrected by a period of fasting, then followed by maintaining a balanced diet. With gallstones, attention is paid initially to a modified fast in conjunction with enemas and hot compresses.

Herbalists have recommended garlic, marigold, and sage among many other treatments in the management of a variety of G.I. disturbances.

Homeopathy considers the patient's personality and constitution to be as important as the symptoms themselves in the management of a given disorder. The remedy is then prepared, having been tailored to the given individual.

Osteopathy and chiropractic cures are based on the principle that proper manipulation of the spine is critical to the integrity of all the organs of the body. As such, G.I. disorders may be related to the spinal defect.

Acupuncture has been used for a wide variety of G.I. ailments in addition to anesthesia, and, as with other alternative forms of therapy, it is geared to the given individual. There are 12 pulses, 6 on each wrist, 1 for each main meridian. These meridians are identified with various organs. Needles are then applied at certain points to restore the balance of "ki energy." Acupuncturists have felt comfortable treating ulcers, diarrhea, constipation, and even colitis.

Naturopaths adhere to the principle that an accumulation of toxic waste materials produced by years of improper living leads to disease. Symptoms of acute illness are manifestations of the body's attempt to rid itself of these toxic products. Enhancement of the body's ability to return to health can occur by fasting, proper diet, general body-building, and proper hygiene. The diet usually consists of 60 percent raw foods, 20 percent unrefined carbohydrates, and 20 percent protein. There may be additions to the diet in the form of cancer-inhibiting enzymes or vitamins.

Emotional stress and depression have long been felt by some to contribute to the development of gastrointestinal disorders, including cancer. Many alternative forms of psychological therapies have been proposed, including visualization therapy, meditation, and atavistic regression. The common denominator in these anticancer therapies is that once a person is free of stress, then homeostatic mechanisms can combat the cancer cells.

As with forms of therapy preferred by mainstream medicine, alternative therapies are directed at a restoration or augmentation of natural forces, which is designed to combat malignancy. The common view is that cancer is a manifestation of death itself. For some reason, be it age, depression, or a lack of touch with one's vital forces, cancer ensues. Therapy revives the vital forces to attack the spread of cancer.

No alternative.therapy should be used alone in the management of cancer. However, any form of therapy that can promote hope and alleviate depression is useful. Visits to healers and healing centers throughout the centuries have also been felt by some to produce cures.

As can be seen from the preceding material, there are many G.I. disorders that can be diagnosed and treated by the patient. The greatest percentage of G.I. symptoms seen by gastroenterologists in patients can be modified significantly by such simple measures as changes in the diet and the cessation of smoking and drinking alcohol. Familiarity by the patient with G.I. symptoms can be particularly helpful to the physician in diagnosing the condition. Oftentimes, reassurance may be all that is necessary in the therapy of the condition.

Also, attempts at behavioral modification may reduce those symptoms that are clearly related to stress.

In those patients with a G.I. disorder that has a potentially high risk of developing complications, a close relationship between the physician and patient should be developed. The individual should be an active participant in his or her care and should be as knowledgeable as possible about the condition. The following societies may provide reading materials:

American Digestive Disease Society, 7720 Wisconsin Avenue, Bethesda, Md. 20014, (301) 652-9293

National Foundation for Ileitis and Colitis Inc., 444 Park Avenue South, New York, N.Y. 10016, (212) 685-3440

American Liver Foundation, 998 Pompton Avenue, Cedar Grove, N.J. 07009, (201) 857-2626

Female Health Care

UROLOGY AND REPRODUCTION

Women can suffer a wide variety of problems and conditions linked to the urological or reproductive systems. Some of these conditions occur naturally and are linked with changes in age or with pregnancy. Others can be prevented by understanding their origins, or the risk factors that can lead to problems. In this section we present a simplified overview of female urologic and reproductive problems, along with information about these systems that every woman should understand. Needless to say, every woman who has reached puberty should be under the care of a physician and see one on a regular basis.

URINARY TRACT INFECTION AND INFLAMMATION

Young women appear to be the most susceptible to urinary tract infections. There is no question that during the life cycle of most females, there occurs some infection or inflammatory condition involving the bladder, especially during early adulthood. Part of this has to do with the fact that the urethra is short in the female, so that organisms can colonize easily in the vagina and infection can be established. The most important piece of news is that in a young, healthy female there is rarely a serious underlying genitourinary disorder.

HOW WE MAKE A DIAGNOSIS

If you develop symptoms of urinary tract inflammation or infection, it is not necessary to undergo many of the tests that were historically performed by urologists over the years, such as kidney X rays and cystoscopic examination of the bladder. The exception to this is the person with a history of urinary tract infections as a child. However, a routine complete urinalysis should be performed when someone develops symptoms such as burning, frequency, urgency, and discomfort on urination. This will determine whether there are signs and symptoms of infection in the urinary tract.

Generally speaking, when there is a bacterial infection present, white cells and red cells are present in great numbers. The appropriate treatment is short-term antibiotics, but a urinalysis and culture should be obtained to make sure that the infection actually has gone away.

If the urinary tract infection is cleared easily, it is not necessary to consider other forms of treatment or diagnostic studies. If the condition recurs with bacterial infection on a number of occasions, bacterial suppressive therapy, such as with Bactrim or Septra or their generic equivalents, is the treatment of choice, rather than embarking on further diagnostic studies. Three to six months of therapy will generally prevent most recurring urinary tract infections in susceptible females. During this period the infection will stop and the antibiotic therapy can be discontinued after the three- to six-month period. Most women will not develop recurring infection after this period of time.

There are many women who have symptoms of urinary infection, but the urinalysis and culture don't show it. These are women for whom stress generates symptoms in the bladder and urethra. When diagnostic studies are performed, no anatomic abnormalities can be found. Susceptible patients in this group have their urinary tract symptoms aggravated by coffee, tea, alcohol, cold weather, spicy foods, or anxiety-producing situations. These patients do not require antibiotic therapy because there is no infection present. Generally speaking, fluid restriction, antispasmodics, hot tub baths, and avoidance of the irritants listed above will prevent their symptoms.

PREMATURE PUBERTY

Premature puberty presents many different and unexpected urologic and gynecologic changes in young women. If a girl starts to undergo development of the breasts or menstrual periods at age 6, for example, it's possible that this may be related to a tumor. On the other hand, it may be related just to premature puberty, and no identifiable cause found.

If at all possible one should try to delay the first signs of premature puberty. Obviously the young girl won't be emotionally ready for it. At the same time, of course, none of her friends are having menstrual cycles. She may have an initial growth spurt, followed by no further growth. Thus her adult height may be less than expected. For premature puberty unrelated to tumor, it is possible to delay it with a drug. But this is currently experimental.

MENSTRUATION

Just as potentially serious as premature puberty is delayed menstruation—that is, if a woman has not had her menstrual period by age 16 or certainly age 18. The average age of menstrual onset is 13.

In order for menstruation to occur, a woman must have an adequately functioning hypothalamus (part of the brain), pituitary gland, ovary, and uterus that is capable of responding to these hormonal releases, and an opening out to the vagina so that a response can occur. Not only does there have to be normal interaction between these various parts for this interaction to occur, but one also has to have a normal psychological state, normal weight, normal thyroid, and normal adrenal function.

If a woman has not had a period by age 18, it is labeled primary amenorrhea. This is usually related to problems she was born with, including absence of the uterus or the vagina, or, for example, maldevelopment or nondevelopment of the ovaries.

SYMPTOMS OF AMENORRHEA

In order to understand amenorrhea, think of it in terms of "compartments": the hypothalamus, pituitary, ovary, or uterus.

Drugs that can cause amenorrhea are sometimes the major tranquilizers, such as thorazine.

Sheehan's postpartum necrosis can cause amenorrhea; it occurs because of excessive bleeding at the time of childbirth and if the pituitary ceases to function.

In addition, pituitary tumors can result in amenorrhea; they are usually ones that secrete prolactin. These tumors are not usually lifethreatening, but they certainly can produce amenorrhea and, subsequently, infertility.

Ovarian causes of amenorrhea could be the result of cysts, which produce increased amounts of androgens or estrogens. The classic condition is polycystic ovary syndrome, which causes amenorrhea as well as hirsutism, sometimes associated with obesity. It is thought to result from abnormal stimulation from the hypothalamus and pituitary to the ovary.

Other conditions involving the ovary may be premature ovarian failure and premature menopause.

One uterine cause of amenorrhea could be a congenital condition in which the uterus doesn't develop at all. A more common adult condition is Asherman's syndrome, caused by damage to the endometrium and usually related to a D&C associated with a pregnancy. When there is destruction of the endometrium, it is incapable of responding to the estrogen and progesterone of the ovary. That is, all the hormones have been produced in adequate quantities but there is no endometrium capable of responding or being sloughed off.

As far as problems related to interactions between the various "compartments," one should keep in mind a common condition that is becoming more and more common: excessive weight loss. This may be associated with anorexia nervosa, bulimia, or weight loss on an extreme diet. When a woman has fallen below a critical weight, amenorrhea can frequently develop.

The long-term health implications of this type of amenorrhea are not known. There are some suspicions that it may be associated with the development of osteoporosis later in life. On the other hand, if one is exercising a great deal, it is known that exercise will have a preventive effect as far as osteoporosis is concerned. In general with amenorrhea, if it is related to decreased estrogen production, osteoporosis has to be considered.

Excess stress, perhaps associated with extra or too much exercise, may itself be a cause of amenorrhea as well. For amenorrhea that is congenital, such as with the absence of the uterus or vagina, there are no good therapies. One can surgically try to create a functioning vagina, so that the woman will be capable of having sexual relations. For conditions that are iatrogenic, such as Asherman's syndrome, surgery may be of help.

EXCESS MENSTRUATION

When a woman has excess bleeding at the time of menstruation, there are a number of possible reasons. Again one has to think of the reproductive system in terms of compartments.

There could be fibroid tumors in the lining of the uterus. Usually when the fibroids, known as submucosal fibroids, are under the lining of the uterus, a woman will experience heavy bleeding at the time of her period. Usually these fibroids are not associated with bleeding between menstrual cycles. With this heavy bleeding the woman's hematocrit or blood count may fall excessively. The fibroids, when benign, can sometimes be taken care of surgically either through the cervix in a procedure called hysteroscopy, or through a major operation where one actually cuts into the uterus through a laparotomy incision in the abdominal wall.

A newer form of therapy, and still experimental, would be to use GnRH and use it as a long-acting agonist. This would cause a down regulation of pituitary receptors, and thus very little LH would be produced. Thus, the ovary would not be stimulated, and the woman would be temporarily amenorrheac and menopausal. This causes the fibroids to shrink in size, since they require estrogen for stimulation.

One always has to include cancer as a possible cause of excess bleeding. Whenever there is excess bleeding a physician will obtain a sample of the lining of the uterus, through an endometrial biopsy, to be sure that cancer is not present.

Besides cancer, one could have excess growth of the lining of the uterus, which occurs when the ovary produces excess quantities of estrogen. Ultimately the lining of the uterus will outgrow its blood supply, resulting in irregular bleeding. It is typically painless and may be bright red in color. It may be so excessive that the woman will have to come to the hospital because of hemorrhage. But it can usually be treated with progesterone, after one has ruled out the possibility of cancer with an endometrial biopsy.

The times of life when women see this excess bleeding are usually either at the onset of menstruation, which is around age 13 or so, or at the other extreme, around age 50, at the onset of menopause. It is at these times that ovulation becomes least efficient. This is due to the fact that the woman may be producing estrogen without undergoing ovulation. Thus, she does not produce estrogen and progesterone in the usual sequence. The endometrium may thus undergo excess stimulation. This is what may result in dysfunctional uterine bleeding. Treatment would be directed toward the addition of progesterone to stimulate the ovulation. This would in turn prevent endometrial hyperplasia from developing, because of unopposed estrogen stimulation.

DYSMENORRHEA AND OTHER PROBLEMS ASSOCIATED WITH THE MENSTRUAL CYCLE

When a woman is menstruating one of the symptoms frequently associated with this is painful periods. These are cramps that women experience in the lower portion of the abdomen, which may radiate down their legs or up the abdomen. These cramps may be so severe that a woman may have to spend the time in bed, missing school or work. These are real phenomena and are usually related to the release of prostaglandins, which may cause contractions. This problem, called "primary dysmenorrhea," is a natural physiological phenomenon. It has been discovered that if you can inhibit the growth or formation of the prostaglandins you can decrease the pain associated with periods. This principle was behind the advent of antiprostaglandin or prostaglandin synthetase inhibitors. Drugs such as Motrin have been rather effective in the treatment of dysmenorrhea.

On the other hand, there may be a condition called "secondary dysmenorrhea." Secondary dysmenorrhea is the pain associated with the period that has an organic cause. A physician should always look for an organic cause first as a possibility to explain the dysmenorrhea; after one has ruled out an organic cause, then the diagnosis of primary dysmenorrhea is made.

The most common cause of secondary dysmenorrhea is endometriosis. This is the condition that occurs when the lining of the uterus is present in places outside of the uterus: in the Fallopian tubes, in the ovaries, or in the pelvis. This lining responds, theoretically, to the natural hormone production of the woman. Since this is occurring instead when the woman is having her period, the endometrium releases blood into the general peritoneal cavity. Of course, having blood in a foreign place would result in severe pain. This may ultimately go on to form scar tissue.

If endometriosis is the source of the pain, it can be identified by means of laparoscopy. Laparoscopy is a small surgical procedure, usually done under a general anesthesia but possible under a local one, in which an incision is made in the umbilicus and an instrument is inserted into the peritoneal cavity. Laparoscopy is not without risk, but in the hands of a skilled physician, it is relatively safe. Endometriosis can then be identified.

Nobody knows the exact cause of endometriosis. One major cause includes the fact that there is retrograde menstruation—that is, when the woman is having her period, some of the endometrium escapes through the Fallopian tubes into the peritoneal cavity. Another cause includes the fact that there is just a change in the normal lining of the peritoneal cavity, in which it is converted into endometrium and responds to estrogen and progesterone.

Currently, the best way to treat endometriosis, if it is not extensive enough to require surgery, is with drug therapy. What one tries to do is to turn off the ovarian production of hormones. Then, hopefully, there won't be any estrogen or progesterone to increase the endometriosis or to continue forcing it to grow.

Drug therapy for endometriosis is not without side effects. Drugs include oral contraceptives given in a continuous fashion so that the woman doesn't have withdrawal bleeding. Other drugs include Danazol, which is an androgen-type agent used to turn off ovarian production of hormones.

Another condition associated with the menstrual cycle that is obtaining much more visibility in our society now is premenstrual tension syndrome or PMS. A woman suffering from PMS may have a series of symptoms such as: headache, irritability, anxiety, insomnia, and excessive weight gain a number of days prior to menstruation. These symptoms tend to disappear after the menstrual cycle begins.

No one knows the exact reason for the development of PMS but physicians ought to be sensitive to it. It usually occurs in this cyclic fashion, and the physician usually does not make the diagnosis unless he has prior experience. Because the etiology is unknown, therapy for it is even less well known.

Therapies that have been tried but not necessarily proven to be effective include: a diet that avoids salt-containing substances, diuretics, prolactin-inhibiting substances, exercise, and tranquilizers. Progesterone vaginal suppositories as well have been tried, but with varied results.

FEMALE INFERTILITY

About 15 percent of couples in the United States have problems related to infertility. This number will grow as women postpone childbearing by using contraceptive agents. It is theoretically possible that some of these contraceptive agents can produce disease that will ultimately result in infertility.

At the very same time, as women age, their chances increase for developing diseases—endometriosis, for one—which in itself could be a cause for infertility. Finally, with aging itself there is decreased fertility potential. In order to understand how infertility develops, one has to be clear about how pregnancy takes place. It begins very simply with ejaculated sperm traveling through the cervical mucus, up the uterus, and up the Fallopian tubes. Theoretically the ovaries release an egg once a month, and the egg is picked up by the Fallopian tube. Fertilization takes place in the outer third of the Fallopian tube, and it takes about five to seven days for the fertilized egg to travel down the Fallopian tube and end up in the uterine cavity.

If this complicated procedure is what it takes to produce a pregnancy, any abnormality along the way could result in infertility. For example, the husband may not have a good enough sperm count or the sperm may not survive inside the cervical mucus (see Chapter Eighteen). The female's Fallopian tubes may be blocked, the tubes themselves may have adhesions around them which may interfere with tubal motility, or the ovaries may not release eggs.

FERTILITY TESTS

In order to identify where the problem is, one has to do tests. It must be emphasized that infertility is a couple problem, and not a female or a male problem. With some couples, the husband may be able to produce a pregnancy with another woman, and vice versa, the woman may be able to produce a pregnancy with another man; but together they cannot. It is necessary for the physician to isolate where the problem is. Usually doctors start with a sperm count obtained after masturbation. A sperm count should be ideally greater than 20 million per cc. The presence of live sperm in the cervical mucus can be measured through a postcoital test. This would imply that the husband has an adequate sperm count, that the couple is certainly having sexual relations, or that the woman may have antibodies that are killing off her husband's sperm.

We can identify whether or not the Fallopian tubes are open by doing a hysterosalpingogram (an X ray of the uterus and Fallopian tubes), which would confirm patent tubes. If there is any doubt of this, it could be followed up by the surgical procedure known as laparoscopy, which would identify whether the tubes were patent. Dye would be placed through the uterus, and then through the laparoscope, you could see if the dye was coming out through the Fallopian tubes.

Ovulation is detected by indirect methods. There is no perfect proof of ovulation other than if the woman gets pregnant. The indirect methods rely on the following: the fact that when the egg is released the corpus luteum produces progesterone. Progesterone itself may have an effect on the hypothalamus, such that it elevates basal body temperature, and at the same time progesterone could make the endometrium or the lining of the uterus become secretory in nature.

One indirect means of diagnosing ovulation is by a basal body temperature chart, which measures ovulation occurring a day or two prior to the temperature rise. Another means of detecting ovulation would be to obtain ultrasound monitoring and observe the growth of the follicle. Then one can see by ultrasound that the follicle disappears on the day of ovulation. A newer form of ovulation detection would also be obtained by tests that the woman could do at home by adding various reagents to the urine. Then one can see a color change on the day prior to ovulation, when the LH surge occurs.

After one has identified which "compartment" has the problem, it is then possible to form a treatment plan. For example, if the husband's sperm count is low, then one may attempt therapy for the male, but in general, drug therapy for male factor infertility has been disappointing. When the count is very low and nothing can be done to help the male, one may attempt pregnancy by an artificial insemination donor. This should be done by highly reputable physicians to ensure the quality and the background of the donor. There may also be a need for an infertile couple to seek psychological counseling during this process. It's important to consider this aspect of complementary treatment when you approach any infertility specialist.

Surgery for infertility has been disappointing for the most part, which has been the impetus for the development of in vitro fertilization. In vitro fertilization is a technique in which eggs are harvested, usually through laparoscopy but at times with ultrasound guidance. The eggs are incubated in the laboratory with sperm obtained from the husband. After fertilization is complete, the fertilized eggs are transferred back into the uterus of the woman. Currently the success rate of this procedure runs around 20 percent and is very expensive to perform. A newer technique for in vitro fertilization for the couple with unexplained infertility involves the GIFT procedure. This involves obtaining the eggs at time of laparoscopy and then placing them back into the Fallopian tube along with the husband's sperm. Thus, the process of incubation of the sperm and the eggs is avoided. This is ideally used for the couple where no cause for the infertility is evident.

If the problem is identified as inadequate ovulation, one can attempt ovulation induction. Some of the ovulation induction agents include Clomiphene and Perganol. When indicated, these are highly successful forms of therapy. However, it must be emphasized that there is a major risk of hyperstimulation of the ovary. This means that the ovaries can get very enlarged, to the point where if a cyst is present, it could rupture; surgery would then be necessary and part or an entire ovary could be lost. The more common complications of these drugs include, of course, multiple pregnancies. When there are a large number of babies born in one pregnancy, the doctor usually inquires about the use of ovulation-inducing agents. (If success has been obtained with reversing infertility or a couple desires pregnancy, the next thing that could occur, of course, is pregnancy.)

CONTRACEPTION

The flip side of an infertility problem is an unwanted pregnancy. So when a couple begins to have sexual relations, clearly one of their most important concerns is choice of a contraceptive. Unfortunately, it appears in our society that the major burden of contraception is placed on women. The contraceptive agent that has made a major impact on the sexual revolution in our country has been oral contraceptives, The Pill.

THE PILL

The basis for oral contraceptives is that they contain both estrogen and progesterone. This combination tends to have a negative feedback in the hypothalamus and pituitary such that normal gonadotrophins influencing the ovary are decreased. With the decrease, there is no stimulation of the ovary to mature an egg.

Oral contraceptives are not without risk. The major risks include the development or potential development of strokes or myocardial infarcts. These tend to occur more in women over age 35 and especially in women who are smokers. A woman who smokes should not use oral contraceptives after age 35.

There has been no good evidence that oral contraceptives increase the risk of cancer. In fact, if anything they tend to diminish the risk of endometrial cancer. Other benefits of oral contraceptives, besides the fact that they are practically 100 percent effective against pregnancy, is that oral contraceptives may reduce the incidence of pelvic inflammatory disease. They may set up a barrier to prevent this particular risk. Some women do not like taking oral contraceptives because they don't like taking medication. On the other hand, they appear to be quite effective for younger women and certainly are the first line of contraception.

Oral contraceptives are also rather convenient and generally provide little interference with a normal sexual life. In fact, if anything, oral contraceptives tend to become safer as the dose of the hormones in the oral contraceptives are reduced. However, there will be a fine line below which one will not be able to reduce the level of hormones to minimize the risk. As one gets to too low a dose, breakthrough bleeding may ensue. Also, too low a dose would reduce the efficacy of the contraceptive.

Injectible progesterone-alone agents can be used as contraceptives, but the latter is not currently approved for use in the United States. It might be effective for people who have difficulty remembering to take pills. One of the problems with these injectable forms of steroids is that one has to wait some time before the hormone levels decline. This can be associated with a side effect such as bleeding.

IUDs

The next most effective contraceptive is the intrauterine device. It is thought that this works by producing a reaction in the endometrium so that the implanted egg will not produce a pregnancy. The IUD has a problem in that it may be associated with heavier bleeding during periods. It may be associated with dysmenorrhea as well. It is not 100 percent effective against pregnancy, as a small percentage of women will become pregnant.

If pregnancy results, the IUD should be removed at the first sign. If the woman remains pregnant with the IUD in place, a severe infection may develop. If the woman gets pregnant with an IUD in place, there is a possibility of the development of a pregnancy in the Fallopian tube.

Some IUDs are thought to be worse than others as far as infections are concerned, especially if there is a multifiliment string coming out of the IUD. These include the Dalkon Shield, which was removed from the market after being linked to serious injuries and deaths. Other companies have also stopped manufacturing the IUD despite the fact that newer IUD forms have been developed. These are copper-containing IUDs, which are smaller and less symptomatic. Their drawback is that they have to be changed every two to three years.

At this time, the future of this form of contraceptive is very much up in the air. Since studies have shown that the IUD could produce infertility by causing scarring in and around the Fallopian tubes, most IUDs are not currently available in the U.S. The only one in 1986 that one can still prescribe is the Progestasert. However, it is strongly advised that an IUD not be given to any woman who has not had any children.

BARRIER CONTRACEPTIVES

The most popular barrier form of contraception is the diaphragm. This is relatively safe and quite helpful in terms of preventing sexually transmitted infection. Some women do not like to use it for aesthetic reasons. Also, if a woman is sexually active and has intercourse more than twice in six hours, she has to put in more cream. In addition, the woman has to keep the diaphragm in after intercourse. This is uncomfortable for some women, and it is associated with urinary tract infections.

Other forms of barrier contraception range from the contraceptive sponges to foams to spermicidal cream. All of these have drawbacks due to aesthetic reasons and may hamper one's sexual style. They are relatively safe, but they are not 100 percent effective against pregnancy. If one does not use a contraceptive agent that is absolutely effective, then pregnancy may ensue. Another thing to note about these foams and creams is that they all basically contain the same active spermicidal ingredient. The form and method of administration is critical to how a product works and how the user feels when using it.

Another important fact to remember when buying contraceptives is that most forms have both a laboratory effectiveness rating and a use effectiveness rating. The latter is always lower. And this is the indicator that one should go by because it is more closely related to whether a contraceptive works or does not. Almost any form of contraceptive, from the condom to a foam, can be highly effective if the users are motivated to use them *absolutely correctly*. But, in general, most people don't follow instructions that precisely. So remember, the type of contraceptive you choose can be effective only if you want it to be effective.

ABORTIONS

As a generalization, the earlier one has an abortion, the safer it is as far as the woman is concerned. It is best to do them between six to eight weeks, and definitely prior to twelve weeks. The earlier one does it, the less one has to worry about bleeding. The main complications of therapeutic abortions include the possibility of not removing all the tissue. If one doesn't, then the patient could end up with an infection and subsequent infertility. One could have extra heavy bleeding as well because of the retained pregnancy.

STERILIZATION

When a woman has reached a particular age where she feels that her family is complete—this age varies for everybody—then one of the options for her husband to consider is permanent sterilization. The simplest of course is the vasectomy, but some men don't want to have this procedure done.

The woman may then opt herself to have permanent sterilization. This is usually produced by doing a laparoscopy or by electrocauterization of the Fallopian tubes. One can also place a clip or a ring around the Fallopian tubes. Sterilizations can also be done by surgically removing these tubes. This is sometimes done right after a delivery. Sterilizations can even be done by hysterectomy. This is an excessive measure and currently rarely used as a form of sterilization.

When considering a sterilization, a woman has to be really sure that her family is complete. If the woman insists on a sterilization and is rather young, she should consider a sterilization that is potentially reversible. Current therapies allow a reversal of a sterilization, using microsurgical techniques to reconstruct the Fallopian tubes. The success rate is not 100 percent; it is closer to 50 to 60 percent.

PREGNANCY

Pregnancy is a beautiful experience for a woman who desires it. It should be thought of as a natural physiological condition, for it is not an illness. At the same time women and their physicians should be on the lookout for disease processes that could accompany pregnancy, because there is a certain maternal mortality that goes along with it. The problems associated with pregnancy can be divided up into trimesters.

First Trimester

When pregnancy is diagnosed some of the complaints that women may experience include fatigue, nausea, and vomiting. In the past, nausea and vomiting could be treated with antiemetic agents but these have not been considered to be safe lately. The nausea and vomiting of early pregnancy, called hyperemesis gravidarum, or morning sickness, can be so severe that some women are admitted to the hospital; it is important to be sure that a woman does not get dehydrated.

One of the more worrisome complaints that occurs during the first trimester is vaginal bleeding. About 20 to 25 percent of pregnancies terminate in a spontaneous miscarriage. If one has bleeding and cramping and passes tissue, this is usually a sign of miscarriage.

Whenever a woman becomes pregnant, it is important that her physician ensures that it is not an ectopic pregnancy, because this is life-threatening.

This does not necessarily imply that every woman ought to have an ultrasound examination to check her when she is pregnant, as the safety of ultrasound has not been totally confirmed. However, when an ectopic pregnancy is suspected, an NIH consensus conference has suggested that ultrasound is certainly indicated, so it ought to be done.

One important sign of an ectopic pregnancy is to watch for vaginal bleeding, pelvic mass, and pelvic pain. If diagnosis is made soon enough, in the hands of a skilled doctor, the ectopic pregnancy can be removed with a laparoscope; thus a major operation can be avoided.

Second Trimester

The second trimester is sometimes the best part of pregnancy because that is when women feel best and the symptoms of fatigue and morning sickness are gone. Pregnant women feel most active during this particular time and usually have very few medical problems. But women sometimes may suffer miscarriage usually due to a uterine abnormality. If a woman miscarries or has repeated miscarriages, her doctor has to keep this in mind. A hysterosalpingogram is used to identify the outline of the uterus. If the hysterosalpingogram shows an abnormal uterus, then surgery to unify the uterus could be helpful. These procedures usually have a 70 percent success rate.

On the other hand, the miscarriage could be related to the fact that the cervix undergoes premature dilation. In that particular situation a suture placed across the cervix in the second trimester can be used to prevent premature dilation.

One of the more serious complications of the second trimester is premature labor. When labor occurs prior to 37 weeks of pregnancy, it can have serious sequelae both for the infant as well as the mother. Instead of having premature labor, one can have premature rupture of the membranes which surround the infant. This would result in the fluid loss and perhaps loss of barrier to infection. In most cases, in these situations, the mothers go on to have early labor, again, prematurity is one of the serious complications and attempts should be made to prevent it and treat it early.

Third Trimester

In the third trimester conditions associated with pregnancy can be preexisting medical complications that the woman brings into the pregnancy. For example, if she has high blood pressure, this tends to get worse in the third trimester. At the same time, if she has had diabetes, the pregnancy may affect the diabetes and vice versa. Pregnant women who are diabetic must have close control of their diabetes. If they haven't had good control of blood sugar in the first trimester then there is an increased incidence of birth defects.

If a woman has had congenital heart disease and is pregnant, this can produce increased stress on her heart. Consultation with a cardiologist would be helpful in terms of keeping the woman's cardiovascular status stable.

Diseases specifically associated with pregnancy in the third trimester include preeclamptic toxemia. In this particular condition the woman develops high blood pressure as a result of pregnancy; there is a peculiar renal lesion, and the woman has proteinuria and edema as well as weight gain. The only treatment for preeclamptic toxemia is delivery. This combination of high blood pressure, protenuria, and edema, if left untreated, may proceed to the point where the woman develops full-blown seizures.

This is one condition in which an obstetrician can certainly make a difference. With intervention and close monitoring of the pregnancy you can prevent the full-blown development of this problem, which would have serious implications both for the mother and for the child.

In some cases when the pregnancy is not proceeding well, the baby may not get adequate oxygen and may undergo growth retardation. Some of the problems associated with inadequate oxygen for the baby could be determined by a biophysical profile. This is ultrasound monitoring of the baby to make sure that it has good activity and good growth, at the same time measuring fetal heart rate to make sure that it has good variability and that there is no deceleration, especially after a spontaneous contraction of the uterus. A spontaneous contraction of the uterus followed by a fall in the heart rate usually implies a late deceleration, which indicates poor oxygenation of the fetus.

Other specific problems associated with pregnancy in the third trimester could be related to the placenta. For example, if the placenta prematurely separates from the uterus one has placenta abruption. This could be life-threatening for both the mother and the baby because it can be followed by hypertension and other problems, like severe pelvic pain. On the other hand, painless vaginal bleeding in the third trimester is usually related to placenta previa, where the placenta precedes the baby. In this particular condition, obviously, the baby cannot come through first, and a Caesarean section is mandatory.

BIRTH

As far as delivery is concerned, there is either a Caesarean section or a vaginal delivery. The major indications for "C section" include both maternal and fetal problems. Fetal indications occur if monitoring the baby shows decreased ability to tolerate labor. Maternal indications would be such that it is not in the mother's interest to have labor. This could be related to a mother being very sick, and not being allowed to labor for 8–10 hours. Another indication could be if the mother had an operation on her uterus, where the endometrial cavity was opened, it could then be thought that the uterus would not be able to tolerate the stress of labor.

Inadequate oxygenation of the baby during labor is measured both by monitoring of the fetal heart rate as well as by measuring pH, which is done by obtaining a fetal scalp sample. If the doctor finds this problem, it is critical to have the baby delivered as quickly as possible by Caesarean section.

Fortunately, most deliveries are accomplished uneventfully and again can be an exciting experience for everybody involved, including the health care provider. It is estimated that in only 20 percent of pregnancies is there some problem for which intervention by an obstetrician will be necessary.

Following delivery, one has to decide whether or not to circumcise the male infant. It is done in some religious groups, and other people feel it should be done for cleanliness. This is a controversial matter, as some pediatricians feel that doing a circumcision is not necessary for future cleanliness or decreased cancer incidence.

As far as breastfeeding is concerned, not only can this be a positive aesthetic experience and help in the bonding of mother and child, but there is some good evidence to show that antibodies pass through the mother's breast milk that could prevent infections in the newborn infant. Specifically these antibodies prevent gastrointestinal infections.

After delivery, one again has to be concerned with the use or nonuse of contraception as described earlier.

MENOPAUSE

As women age, the ovary eventually runs out of follicles. This usually occurs at about age 50. With the lack of estrogen a number of problems may arise. Women may experience vasomotor flushes, or hot flashes. These are not life-threatening in nature but can be very disturbing to any woman. These are real phenomena that can be measured objectively. They occur during the day as well as at night. They are initially felt as an objective sensation, which is then followed by peripheral vasodilation; the woman feels warm and then begins to sweat as her body temperature comes down.

Postmenopausal women also have vaginal dryness. This is due to the lack of estrogen. The woman may experience pain with intercourse upon entry. This condition usually responds well to estrogen replacement therapy. Another medical condition that is very common for postmenopausal women, and is certainly of major public health impact, is osteoporosis (see Chapter Fifteen). It occurs much more frequently in women than men. It is frequently responsible for hip fractures at a later age, and is responsible for many of the deaths in our society. The addition of estrogen replacement therapy and calcium, as well as exercise, have been shown to be helpful in slowing osteoporosis.

The women most at risk for osteoporosis are white, slender women who smoke. Using objective measurements to detect bone density, a physician can identify who is at risk for osteoporosis and then advise that particular individual to be treated.

While we do know that estrogen replacement therapy can reduce the loss of bone mass in women going through menopause, the evidence that estrogen prevents heart disease in postmenopausal women is still controversial and we need more data. The risks of estrogen replacement therapy include the potential of developing endometrial cancer. It appears though that if one adds a progestin to estrogen, this risk of endometrial cancer is greatly reduced. The evidence of estrogen causing breast cancer is still controversial; some studies have suggested it, but most have not.

Using estrogen is an individual decision for a woman in menopause. She has to weigh the benefits and risks of hormone replacement therapy against the risk of osteoporosis and decide for herself. This is a decision that should be made in consultation with her physician as she enters menopause.

CANCERS OF THE REPRODUCTIVE SYSTEM

A lot of the cancers associated with the female reproductive system can be diagnosed rather early if the physician and the patient are aware of them. If the patient goes regularly for routine care and is educated as to what particular signs and symptoms to look for, most cancers can be diagnosed early. Of course, the earlier the diagnosis, the earlier the stage of the disease, the better the chance that therapy will work for that particular individual.

Cancer of the Cervix

This is one disease that can clearly be prevented if a woman is very careful about going to see her physician regularly for exams, especially the Pap smear. Prior to the cervix undergoing cancerous change, a number of changes occur in the cells. The cells may go from atypical to dysplasia to, finally, full-blown cancer. If a woman has a Pap smear once a year, an early indication of cell change could be obtained.

If the Pap smear identifies abnormal cells, this could be followed up by culposcopically directed biopsies. The culposcope magnifies the cervix and any abnormal areas would be biopsied. Once these areas are identified, the condition, if premalignant, could be treated either with surgical removal, freezing of the cervix, laser therapy, or even hot cauterization of the cervix. In this particular way a major cancer could be avoided, while still "precancerous."

Usually cancer of the cervix tends to occur in women who have had intercourse at a young age or start having children at a young age, and also in women who have had HPV (human papilloma virus) infections. If it is not diagnosed early enough, the treatment may vary from radical surgery to radical hysterectomy to radiation therapy. The later the stage at which it's diagnosed, the less success there is likely with therapy.

Endometrial Cancer

Endometrial cancer tends to occur in women in their fifties and sixties, and more often in obese women. It is felt that endometrial cancer is preceded by a "precancerous hyperplasia." It is thought to be related to excess estrogen; thus any woman who is producing lots of estrogen would be at risk for it. It tends to occur in women who are overweight because they have peripheral conversion, which means some of their male hormones from their adrenal gland and ovaries convert to estrogen. It is felt that they don't have enough progesterone to counteract the estrogen, and are thus unovulatory.

The major sign of this is abnormal vaginal bleeding. Usually if one has the first symptoms the doctor could make the diagnosis relatively early and treat the woman before it developed to full-blown cancer. If the bleeding signifies hyperplasia, that could be treated with progesterone. If it signifies early cancer it could be treated with surgery by doing a hysterectomy. If the cancer is further advanced, one may have to add radiation therapy. It's vital to see a physician at the first sign of bleeding.

Vaginal Cancer

Clear cell cancer of the vagina has been seen more often recently, and is usually related to the daughters of mothers who took diethylstilbestrol (DES) during pregnancy. It should thus be stressed that women must not take any hormones during pregnancy unless they are receiving progesterone supplementation. This ought to be carefully documented before it is prescribed. Cancer of the vagina itself is rare.

Vulvar Cancer

This particular cancer usually occurs in older women. It may appear as a little growth of the vulva area. It is important that physicians examine the vulva area carefully and biopsy any abnormal discoloration or abnormal area. The treatment may be rather extensive, usually requiring a radical vulvectomy.

VAGINAL DISCHARGE

Finally, one of the major problems that sends a lot of women to the gynecologist is the development of a vaginal discharge. It is critical that the physician takes a careful history, noting, for example, if the woman has bleeding after intercourse. In this case the doctor has to be sure that cancer of the cervix is not present. Therefore it is important to do a Pap smear at once and make sure there are no vaginal lesions.

On the other hand, the woman may have a purulent discharge. Here it is important to do a lab culture to be sure that gonorrhea is not present. If the discharge is white and cottage cheese-like in appearance, this usually implies a yeast type of infection. With the recurrent yeast type of infection, diabetes is a possibility, because yeast tends to grow and flourish in a high sugar environment. The vaginal discharge should also be examined under the microscope. This may reveal the presence of trichomonas.

SUMMARY

The most important thing is for a woman to be aware of her own body changes. She ought to approach her physician when she notices abnormal things such as vaginal bleeding after intercourse. She ought to be aware of certain family problems, so that if there is a family history of breast cancer, she knows she is more at risk for it.

At the other extreme, certain diseases can be prevented. For example, if a woman has never been pregnant she ought not to have an IUD, because an IUD could be associated with future infertility. Similarly, stopping smoking would be helpful because we know that women who smoke are more at risk for the development of osteoporosis. If the woman is sexually active and she is with a partner that she is not sure of, she ought to approach her physician to have cultures taken to rule out any sexually transmitted diseases. Some of these sexually transmitted diseases can be associated with future medical problems.

By a combination of patient awareness, as well as seeing a physician when any problem ensues, many gynecologic problems can by avoided. Women should also be aware of environmental problems and how they could adversely affect their future health. At the same time, by following a good diet, avoiding certain toxic substances, seeing her physician when necessary, and getting annual exams in which Pap smears are done, a woman should experience a state of good overall health.

Male Urological Conditions

Most men suffer from conditions linked to their urinary systems as they age. Though they are often very painful and annoying, they are frequently simple to treat. Some of these conditions can be overcome by recognizing potential risk factors. In other cases, prompt treatment is the best course of action. In this section we outline in detail some of the more common male urologic conditions.

MALE PROSTATE CONDITIONS

The most common male prostate problem usually occurs when there is an obstruction. Clearly, all men, as they get older, are susceptible to prostatic obstruction, usually a function of age. Most men over the age of 50 who have gradual enlargement of their prostate may or may not have difficulty urinating. But, it's a myth that this means the condition is precancerous; in fact, the majority of men with this enlargement and the symptoms relating to it do not have cancer.

Men with poor-caliber stream and hesitancy, who are getting up a number of times a night, though, need treatment. Unfortunately, there is no medication that can shrink the size of the prostate, and the condition will usually get worse over time, although that time frame is usually indeterminate.

Symptoms

Most important in the assessment of a man with prostate problems are his symptoms. Do the symptoms bother him? Does he mind getting up two or three times a night? Does he mind waiting forty to sixty seconds to complete his urinary stream? Different men have various levels of tolerance for these symptoms.

There are some very simple things that an individual can do to assess how much difficulty he is having voiding urine, and one of these is simply keep track of voiding patterns.

Put a pencil and paper on the back of the toilet and leave it there. Every morning for a week, on arising, void into a large container instead of the toilet. When voiding begins, count the seconds, and when the sustained stream ends, stop counting the seconds. Record the amount of time urination took, then empty the large container into a measuring cup to determine the number of cubic centimeters (cc) voided. By dividing seconds into the volume voided, you can obtain a mean urinary flow rate, which can be compared to that of other males.

The normal rate in the adult male is over 10 cc per second. Therefore, if it takes you thirty seconds to produce 300 cc, you have a normal flow rate. Mild symptoms of obstruction would be in the 7 to 9 cc per second range, moderate in the 4 to 6 cc range. A range of 1 to 3 cc per second is severe and suggestive of severe outlet obstruction. This test can be repeated every four to six months. If there is a diminishing of the rate, then one should be in the care of a urologist.

We can't make a diagnosis that the patient has a prostate condition (or some other form of obstruction such as a scar or stricture) on the basis of flow rates alone. However, most patients have a reduction in their urinary flow rates because of a gradual enlargement of the prostate. If they have symptoms that are getting worse, it's important that they are examined by a urologist, or by a physician who is experienced in performing rectal examinations and especially in assessing the prostate. What's important to the urologist is not so much the size of the prostate, but whether or not there is a change in its consistency. Also, a nodule that is hard would suggest a malignancy that would be associated with this difficulty in voiding urine.

Of most patients with prostate cancer, about 90 percent can be reassured that they don't have cancer based on the rectal examination alone. Approximately 10 percent will have an incidental prostate cancer found at the time of the prostectomy for benign condition; this just shows that the rectal exam is not 100 percent sure. The blood test called an acid phosphatase can be performed if there is an abnormal rectal exam.

If a patient has difficulty voiding to the point where he is complaining, has poor flow rates but normal urinary sediment, and his prostate does not suggest malignancy, then further diagnostic studies are recommended. An example would be a kidney X ray, which requires the injection of intravenous contrast and a bowel preparation, to determine that the upper urinary tract is normal and to determine if the patient is able to empty his bladder or not.

An alternative to a kidney X ray is the ultrasound examination. This is also a satisfactory screening tool for this particular condition and its advantages are that it is noninvasive, does not require bowel preparation, and does not run the risk of contrast reaction. Both the ultrasound or IVP X ray can be performed on an outpatient basis.

YOUNGER MEN

In the younger age group, under age 50, prostate cancer and prostate obstruction are not a serious problem. More frequently, younger men can have symptoms that are suggestive of urinary tract inflammation. There are three conditions which have similar symptoms but different causes.

BACTERIAL PROSTATITIS

The first condition is true bacterial prostatitis. This is the corollary to the female bacterial urinary tract infection. In this case urinalysis is abnormal, urine cultures confirm an infection and the patient has symptoms such as burning, frequency, and urgency similar to those of a urinary infection in women.

Antibiotics are the treatment of choice here. A screening kidney X ray in a young male will generally confirm that there is no anatomic abnormality, and flow rates are recommended just to rule out lower urinary tract obstruction from a urethral stricture. If the patient has symptoms of infection but the urinalysis culture is negative, then bacterial infection is ruled out and bacterial prostatitis is not the diagnosis.

PROSTATOSIS

When a rectal exam confirms many white cells, the condition is diagnosed as prostatosis. Nonbacterial infections can occur from chlamydial infection, which requires specialized culture techniques. A more pragmatic solution to this condition is treatment with broad-spectrum antibiotics, such as tetracycline or erythromycin; if prostatic symptoms do not clear, further testing is worthwhile. The problem with chlamydial cultures is that they cannot be done quickly and they are quite expensive. Since there is no major hazard to the patient's health, a more prudent solution is to treat the patient after routine culture techniques, and to consider further studies only if the patient's symptoms do not respond.

PROSTATODYNIA

This last condition is similar to a female urethral syndrome. It has all the characteristics of urinary inflammation, but the patient also identifies causative factors such as aggravation or precipitation by coffee, tea, alcohol, cold weather, spicy foods, anxiety, fatigue, etcetera. This condition is called prostatodynia, and in general the treatment involves an antispasmodic, hot tub baths, fluid restriction, and avoidance of those factors that cause irritation.

The precise nature of the cause of prostatodynia is unknown, but it is self-limited, tends to be recurrent, and generally responds to conservative measures. Invasive diagnostic studies such as cystoscopic examination or other therapeutic manipulations are generally costly and do not help in controlling the symptoms of this condition.

TESTICULAR CONDITIONS

Scrotal masses are especially anxiety-producing for the young male patient, who is generally convinced that he has cancer. Fortunately, cancer of the prostate is very rare, and today with modern chemotherapy, adjunctive surgery, and radiation, most can be cured, even in the advanced stage. This is a remarkable development in the field of urology in the past five to seven years, and one of the true triumphs of modern medicine.

Symptoms

Scrotal masses should be divided into two major categories: painful and painless. Cancer of the testicle is a painless condition, although occasionally a hemorrhage can occur and the tumor can produce discomfort. Awareness is an important part of prevention of this disease. Breast self-examination has been around for some time, but only recently has self-examination of the testicles been widely disseminated in lay literature. (See Chapter Thirteen for more information on testicular cancer and self-examination.)

Cancer of the testicle causes enlargement and heaviness of the testicle, but not the surrounding appendages. Examination by a board-certified urologist generally leaves little doubt if there is a problem within the testicle itself. All solid testicular masses should be explored to rule out cancer of the testes.

In the 30 to 40 percent of patients with testicular cancer, blood tests show the presence of alpha feto protein and human chorionic gonadatrophin. These two hormones will be elevated and will be followed throughout the course of diagnosis and treatment. Generally speaking, if the two don't respond with treatment this suggests residual disease and the search should continue until the residual disease is found and treated.

A confirmatory testicular ultrasound exam can be very useful as both a second opinion and for ruling out cystic masses of the testicle and its appendages, which are not malignant. Masses of the testes are generally hydroceles, fluid-filled structures surrounding the entire testes, or spermatoceles, which generally arise from, and are attached to, the upper pole of the testes. Neither one of these conditions require any treatment, except for cosmetic reasons.

Swelling of the testes usually represents an inflammation of the appendage of the testes, called epididymitis. This involves a structure attached to the testes through which the spermatozoa pass on the way to the urinary tract. Most of the time the cause of epididymitis is unknown, but it can be associated with urinary tract infection, especially in the older patient.

Epididymitis can also be caused by retrograde flow of urine down the ejaculatory duct, and is seen especially in weight lifters and parachutists. The condition is not dangerous, but it can cause a significant amount of discomfort of the testes and enlarge it over a number of weeks. Treatment of this condition is with antiinflammatory agents and antibiotics.

OTHER RISKS

The patient with undescended testes is at some risk of testicular cancer. Generally speaking, if a child is born with undescended testes, the testes should be brought down when diagnosed. This means doing repairs on these children at a very young age, generally before the age of 2. This we hope will ensure fertility in that undescended testes. It has been clearly shown by electron microscopy that changes occur in the undescended testes in ages earlier than 3. After six or seven years, the undescended testes is incapable of producing normal spermatozoa. In the true undescended abdominal testes the incidence of malignancy is still small but is forty times that of the patients that have two normally descended testes. In most cases, if the testes was not brought down in childhood, it should be either brought down or removed in adulthood providing that the patient is still young. At approximately 50 to 55 years of age, the risk of developing malignancy in that undescended testes is no greater than that for the normal population.

Fortunately, if this condition has not been corrected by adulthood, simple exploration will be successful to identify where the testes is, and it can be removed on an outpatient basis. However, this will require anesthesia.

Diagnostic studies such as ultrasound and abdominal pelvic CAT scan can be helpful in locating the undescended testes in this latter condition. There is a higher incidence of infertility in patients who have unilateral undescended testes, and this should be taken into account in family planning.

SEXUAL DYSFUNCTION

No urology problem raises more anxiety in the male than that caused by sexual difficulty. There are few true organic or anatomic causes for impotence, or inability to maintain an erection. The known causes of permanent sexual difficulty are: radical prostatectomy or cystectomy for cancer of the prostate or bladder; long-standing diabetes; severe arteriosclerosis; and bowel resection for cancer of the rectum.

However, in general, most patients who have sexual dysfunction have a psychological component to their problem.

Generally, any patient with sexual dysfunction will have a normal desire, and will be able to ejaculate through masturbation, even with a flaccid penis. The most frequent complaint is difficulty achieving and maintaining an erection. If the patient has a history of being able to achieve a good-quality erection with a full bladder, then it is unlikely that there is an anatomic problem, and psychological treatment should be sought with the patient's partner.

A serum prolactin test will rule out a pituitary gland basis for the sexual dysfunction, which is rare. Nocturnal penile tumescence studies are now available as an outpatient procedure, using a *Dacomed* nocturnal penile testing device. Basically, a band is placed around the penis at night, and if three small filaments that hold the device in place are broken, it suggests spontaneous, good-quality erection. This test, while not foolproof, is generally indicative that there is no anatomic abnormality.

Generally speaking, if organic anatomic abnormality is present, a penile prosthesis can be inserted, but it only corrects the erectile function. If ejaculation is not possible, this cannot be corrected by a penile prosthesis. Frequently patients with diabetes are ideally suited for the placement of a penile prosthesis because ejaculatory competence remains normal, even though the disease can cause impotence.

For those patients who are psychologically impotent, counseling should be carried out prior to considering any surgical intervention, since often these causes can be corrected without surgery. When psychological counseling is needed, it is important that the involved couple be treated together whenever possible.

MALE INFERTILITY

Male infertility is a difficult problem to treat from a number of points of view. First of all, the condition of infertility can involve both husband and wife (see Chapter Seventeen on female infertility). It is a highly charged emotional issue, and it requires a great deal of time and effort both on the couple's part and on the part of their physician to resolve. Any couple seeking counseling for infertility should seek a specialist in this area with experience.

The infertile couple should be involved with two physicians: the gynecologist, who has a specialty in infertility, evaluates the wife, and the urologist evaluates the husband. Communication between both the gynecologist and the urologist is critical for the proper assessment and management of this problem. There are excellent support groups which provide information as well. In particular there is RESOLVE, a nonprofit organization with national offices in Belmont, Massachusetts, (617) 484-2424. RESOLVE provides excellent literature and direction for the infertile couple as to where they can obtain professional help in specific areas.

The definition of infertility varies with individuals and is time-related. The couple that is 21 years of age is treated differently from the couple that is 34 years of age and trying to achieve pregnancy. From a urologist's point of view, if a year or two of unprotected intercourse does not result in pregnancy, this generally suggests an infertility problem.

Both the husband and wife should be evaluated completely. For the woman, a careful history and pelvic exam should be carried out as part of her initial evaluation. The husband should have at least two or three qualitative semen analyses. The importance of the quality of semen analyses cannot be overemphasized, so it's important that the tests be carried out by an experienced and competent team.

Patient history as to environmental exposure, radiation, drugs, or major illness over the previous six months is important. A family history of infertility problems or any significant past urological history are also of interest. Careful exam by the urologist is important to assess the size of the testes. A patient with soft testes may have a problem. The presence or absence of the vas deferens, the connecting tube from the testicle to the inguinal canal, is important to assure that the collecting structures can deliver the sperm from the testes to the urinary tract. A prostate exam should be performed to rule out infection or inflammation and to test for the presence of prostatic secretions in a normal urinalysis.

If the patient has a varicocele, which is an enlarged group of dilated veins that surround the testicle and can be easily felt by the examining physician, this may have some significance in evaluating the infertile couple. In general, patients with varicocele should be tested for abnormalities of their semen as well.

The standard of care in the urological community has been that when dealing with an infertile couple with a varicocele problem, one of the options is to perform a varicocelectomy, because this may play a role in the patient's abnormal semen analysis.

If the problem is diagnosed as sperm density and motility, there are many medications available, both by injection and by oral intake. Currently Clomid has been the oral medical treatment of choice. This medication is not approved by the Federal Drug Administration for male infertility (it is approved for females), but is widely used anyway in this country for the treatment of idiopathic oligospermia (low sperm count). One abnormal semen analysis may not be a true reflection of the condition. Multiple semen analyses should be obtained over time, and the patient should be examined and reevaluated.

SUMMARY

In general, male urologic and reproductive problems, like those of women, can be treated effectively if they are caught early enough. Men must not only become aware of changes in their bodies, but they must take action to correct a problem before it's too late. Women are usually involved in a health-care system, since they frequently see a gynecologist, especially after childbirth. Men, however, ignore their urological problems out of fear or embarrassment. This is the reason why most male sexual difficulties become more severe than they need be. Every man must take charge of his own health care and be responsible when his system sends him a message that all is not well. It's a good idea for every man at least to know the name of a good, competent urologist whom he can consult as he reaches middle age, when common problems such as prostate conditions pop up.

SEXUALLY TRANSMITTED DISEASES

Sexually transmitted diseases are a major concern to both men and women today. It's also a field with continually emerging information which can help one in reducing risks. To some extent, beating the odds of an STD requires simple common sense, and some education as to the nature of these diseases. The most common STDs are herpes, syphilis, gonorrhea, chlamydia, and AIDS. For some STDs, like herpes and AIDS, we have little potential "cures," but some hopeful treatments.

Both men and women are at risk for some contagious sexually transmitted diseases. These include viral diseases such as genital herpes. When a woman contracts herpes, she is at increased risk for cervical cancer at a later age, since there is believed to be an association between the development of herpes and cervical cancer.

On the other hand, if a woman first contracts a sexually transmitted disease during pregnancy, there is increased risk of infecting the fetus as it passes through an infected birth canal. It is critically important to obtain cervical cultures in the third trimester to be sure that the woman is not still infected.

One drug, acyclovar, has proven effective against some genital herpes for both men and women. Found under the brand name, Zovirax, it is taken either orally, in a cream form, or by injection. While generally effective, this drug is not to be used by pregnant women, and it has been linked to reduced fertility in men.

Another sexually transmitted disease is chlamydia, which has recently been identified as a cause of pelvic inflammatory disease in women. In itself, chlamydia can produce pelvic inflammatory disease and tubal factor infertility.

In the past, syphilis was the most feared sexually transmitted disease. Syphilis is much less of a problem now because of its excellent response to penicillin. Similarly, gonorrhea was a major concern as a cause of tubal factor infertility. Despite antibiotic treatment, a woman who has had exposure to gonorrhea that includes a high fever and severe abdominal pain still has about a 20 percent chance of subsequent infertility. Thus it is critical to get a prompt diagnosis of gonorrhea and appropriate treatment.

The most feared STD today, with good reason, is AIDS. Medical journals are filled with studies, and newspapers, TV shows, and movies concerning this "new" disease are everywhere.

What is AIDS?

AIDS (Acquired Immune Deficiency Syndrome) is really a spectrum of disease caused by a virus called HTLV-III. Symptoms of the disease are fatigue, swollen lymph glands, and an unusual susceptibility to infections by rare bacteria, fungus, or parasites.

AIDS is actually a much rarer STD in this country than in many others. Because at this point it's always fatal and we don't know its cause, we are quite focused on it. Specifically, AIDS seems to occur in this country in homosexual males, IV drug users, and in people requiring multiple blood transfusions.

Recently research around the world has shown a high degree of AIDS in some heterosexual groups, like female prostitutes.

AIDS is not actually treatable, but its infectious complications are.

Many people fear AIDS more than they should, and this fear has led to reduced blood donations. AIDS seems to be transmitted mainly by intense and perhaps indiscriminate sexual contact, blood transfusion (but *not* blood donation), and frequent IV drug use. Clearly it's spread through homosexual anal intercourse and probably now through heterosexual intercourse in high-risk groups.

Despite misconceptions, AIDS is not transmitted easily—for example, by sharing toilet facilities and food. Studies have shown that family members of AIDS victims do not get the disease despite very close contact. Finally, screening of donor blood products, now done on a regular basis, should reduce the risk of AIDS to the general population.

While AIDS is the focus of our concern about STD, it's important to choose sexual partners carefully and get prompt treatment when any symptoms of STD appear. Early treatment and common sense are the only ways to beat the odds of serious future infertility and the even more serious health effects of sexually transmitted disease.

Diabetes

Some 13 million Americans suffer from diabetes. By careful use of medication, new home self-monitoring, and proper diet, diabetics can beat the odds.

What exactly is diabetes?

Diabetes is a disease characterized by the body's inability to control the level of glucose (sugar) that has been consumed in different forms of food.

There are two types of diabetes:

- Type I, which used to be called juvenile diabetes.
- Type II, which is often called adult-onset diabetes.

The most severe form of diabetes is Type I, and affects about 500,000 people, mostly under the age of 20. In this form of the disease, the pancreas does not produce any insulin at all. Type II is far more common and afflicts some 12 million people, most of middle age and older.

Why do we need insulin?

Insulin is a hormone vital to the use of carbohydrates you consume. Carbohydrates you eat are converted in the body mainly to glucose, which in turn provides energy for bodily functions. The pancreas' insulin takes that glucose and helps the body pass it from the blood into your cells where it's stored and used. Insulin also keeps the level of glucose produced in the body in balance. In effect, insulin keeps your system in check. But it often goes awry in diabetics, whose pancreas no longer functions.

Type I diabetics must take insulin injections properly.

Type II diabetics, on the other hand, are not always dependent on synthetic insulin for survival. In fact, their problem is not that their bodies don't produce insulin, rather that their body's insulin is not doing a good job. One reason is that almost all Type II diabetics are overweight. This affects the levels of sugar in their blood and their overall chemical balance.

Why does diabetes develop? Who is at risk?

Diabetes is one disease where a family history is certainly a strong risk factor. However, it is not the only reason one can become diabetic. Most researchers believe that Type I diabetics have a breakdown in their immune system—called an autoimmune reaction—in connection with some form of attack by an unidentified virus on the pancreas. It is thought that some other genetic factor present at birth may cause some victims to be especially susceptible.

Type II diabetes runs in families; it's also thought that some genetic factor may trigger the development of this form of diabetes.

How do you know if you are diabetic?

Diabetes is often an unannounced condition, especially where Type II is concerned.

For most, the first signs of Type I are weight loss, blurred vision, having to urinate frequently, constant thirst, and sometimes vaginal infections in women.

Most people with Type II diabetes find out about it when they have a regular checkup, because a blood test is the only accurate method of determining the presence of any type of diabetes. These tests include a glucose tolerance test, a fasting blood glucose test, and other similar tests. Once you have been diagnosed as diabetic you will always be diabetic.

Does this mean there's no cure?

Diabetes cannot be cured. However, in almost every case, diabetes can be controlled, and a diabetic may live an entirely normal life.

Type I diabetics devote the most time to their treatment, and most are very much in charge of their own care. Type I diabetics learn to give themselves daily insulin injections and follow a carefully defined diet to help them maintain control of their blood sugar levels. Recently, Type Is have been able to monitor their own blood sugar levels with a home monitoring device. This simple device enables the diabetic to measure blood levels and then adjust the amount of insulin appropriately.

Type I diabetics whose sugar is out of control can suffer ketoacidosis, which can lead to a coma. Most Type Is learn to recognize the signs of a change in their body sugar and take appropriate steps to prevent ketoacidosis.

On the other hand, Type II diabetics are most frequently told to lose weight first, before any other treatment is tried. It's been shown that weight loss can bring blood sugar levels back into proper balance in most cases. In fact, the kind of diet used is also relatively unimportant, as long as the amount of weight lost achieves the desired affect on the blood sugar levels. Some Type IIs who cannot exercise or lose enough weight will be given oral antidiabetic drugs, or even insulin.

What happens when diabetes is out of control?

Diabetics are at greater risk than nondiabetics for developing serious disease, like kidney failure, high blood pressure, and atherosclerosis.

Diabetes also affects the blood supply to different parts of the body in many ways that are not fully understood, especially in tissue near the eyes. Blood vessels in the eyes can burst and cause retinopathy, which may lead to blindness, a very common problem for out-of-control diabetics. Fortunately, new treatments with a laser beam can help prevent or repair the eye damage. Type I diabetics are also at risk for infections on the feet. It's recommended that all diabetics pay very close attention to any sores or irritations in the toes or feet and see a physician immediately if any infection occurs.

Diabetic men have been known to suffer impotence as a result of the disease, even though they have a normal desire for sex (see Chapter Eighteen for further information on male impotence). This problem won't always happen, but it may. It should be considered a natural complication of the disease and it should be treated seriously by your physician.

How can you prevent diabetes?

In many cases, diabetes is inevitable. But if you know that you have a family history, especially of Type II, then you can reduce your risk by keeping your weight under control, exercising, and eating a diet high in fiber. And, if you have any early signs of diabetes, you can reduce risk by seeking an early diagnosis.

Most people are treated first and well by their internist or family physician for diabetes. If you have complicated diabetes, or if your physician does not seem attentive to your needs, you might seek care from a diabetologist. You should try to have your initial diagnosis confirmed by a diabetologist and remain under his or her care. After all, these doctors have a wide range of experience with the disease and its very complicated emotional aspects. A good diabetologist can help parents of young Type I diabetics overcome fear and guilt, which is often present.

It's important to remember that diabetes, especially Type II diabetes, can be found in those with other serious life-threatening problems, such as high blood pressure, heart disease, and kidney disease.

Exercise from a Medical Viewpoint

Almost every person needs a regular exercise program, no matter what their capabilities are at the time, no matter what their conditioning is, no matter what their cardiac risk factor profile or their family history is. And there is an exercise program available to every person, including the handicapped.

Exercise has multiple benefits and many purposes, affecting several organs in a beneficial way. Further, there are both physical and psychological benefits.

First, there are the immediate psychological benefits: exercise in a regular pattern can help many people relieve stress. Workout time is a good time for people to be alone, to think. It is similar to and as beneficial as meditation or deep relaxation. There are no telephones, no other people around to bother you. You can enjoy fresh air and nature, and you derive a great sense of personal satisfaction and fulfillment when participating in a regular way. You can see the immediate physical benefits and feel the effects of a regularly scheduled exercise program. Many people find that a regular exercise program may replace regular psychotherapy and, in fact, there are many psychiatrists who prescribe regular exercise as part of their therapy.

Next, the physical side: Obviously, your organ systems are positively affected by regular exercise. It has been shown to benefit the cardiovascular system in many ways. It slows the pulse rate, thereby allowing the heart to work less frequently minute by minute and day by day.

It decreases blood pressure, causing less strain on the heart and decreasing a well-known cardiac risk factor.

In those who have had a heart attack (myocardial infarction) or those who have congestive heart failure, regular exercise done in a graded supervised fashion has been shown to increase patients' overall well-being and increase their capability of performing physical acts and exercise.

While exercise has not been shown to prevent heart attack or increase one's longevity, it has been well shown to decrease many of the cardiac risk factors. And it *can* help control high blood pressure.

People who have peripheral vascular disease suffer pain when walking due to lack of oxygen to the legs (clodication). This group can also benefit from a regular exercise program, which should increase the blood's flow to the leg's muscles and provide enough oxygen. The accompanying pain is often reduced, and surgery can be avoided. Exercise is also well known to help patients who are obese with weight control. Regular workouts will decrease triglyceride levels and also increase high-density lipoprotein (HDL) cholesterol, the so-called "good" cholesterol.

A regular exercise program can decrease one's "fasting blood sugar" and improve one's glucose tolerance in those with juvenile diabetes and with borderline diabetes. Diabetic patients may require less insulin or be able to stop therapy after beginning and sustaining a regular exercise program.

Exercise also decreases one's urge to smoke, thereby controlling one of the most important cardiac risk factors.

People who exercise regularly will frequently adjust their diet, eating less fats, and less heavy protein meals; they will also increase carbohydrate intake.

WHAT IS REGULAR EXERCISE?

When we talk about regular exercise, we are talking about at least three to four exercise periods per week which last twenty to thirty minutes. This causes a sustained increased heart rate and respiratory rate. We usually tell people that they need to work up a sweat or they are not really exercising.

Many people say, "Well, I walk a lot at work," or "I exercise a lot during the day at my job."

For most people this is not enough. If exercise at work was sufficient, most people's risk factors would already be low, their weight would be good, and they would have good physical stamina. Almost all of us need an exercise program in addition to whatever work-related exercise one is doing.

Although the hazards of exercising are minimal in most people, it is important to go into a regular exercise program using the brain as well as the body. A regular exercise program should be initiated in a sane, rational, well-planned-out way; the risks can then be minimized.

Muscular-skeletal discomfort, of course, is the most likely hazard of regular exercise, ranging anywhere from muscle strains to sprains to ruptured ligaments, stress fractures, and actual severe bone fractures among people who engage in dangerous exercise. To avoid injury, start out slowly, build up gradually, and take rest days. Do vigorous exercise one day and rest the next. This doesn't mean you can't exercise at all, but by decreasing exercise levels and resting the body's bones and joints, the risks of muscular-skeletal pain can be minimized.

Most people, however, who do involve themselves in some sort of regular exercise over the years will suffer minor muscular-skeletal injuries (strains or sprains), which can be corrected with rest and adequate preexercise or other stretching and preventive measures.

WHAT ARE THE HAZARDS OF EXERCISE?

One commonly reported danger is sudden death. Sudden death can occur from exercise but, again, in most people, it can be prevented and should, hopefully, be an extremely rare problem. Sudden death is prevented by having a good physical examination prior to beginning any exercise program. This is especially true of anyone who is over age 35 or who has been sedentary for many, many years. A complete physical examination that includes a cardiogram and possibly an exercise tolerance test will ensure that you have no significant cardiac disease that would put you at high risk or sudden death. Sudden death occurs from heart attack (myocardial infarction), or from *dysrhythmia* (irregular beating of the heart). This is especially true in people who get severely dehydrated, low in potassium, or have a primary heart problem.

Sudden death may also occur if someone vomits during strenuous exercise and inhales the vomit into the lungs.

Sometimes exercise can cause blood or protein in the urine, which may be due to a slight lack of oxygen or trauma to the kidneys and the bladder. This is usually not a significant problem. However, people who do get severely dehydrated can suffer kidney failure.

Other risks of regular exercise are as follows:

Since blood pressure and heart rate rise normally during exercise, undue strain on the heart can cause angina or heart attack.

Weather can also lead to injury. A major problem that develops with exercise in many climates throughout the United States and the world is heat and the risk of dehydration. This can certainly be prevented by dressing wisely, by using light-colored clothing, wearing a hat on a hot day, and, most important, drinking adequate amounts of water. Water should be consumed prior to, during, and after long exercise. Don't allow yourself to become thirsty, and make sure that you are always sweating. This allows your temperature regulation mechanisms to continue, preventing severe heat stroke. Heat is a very serious problem for those exercising during the summer and in hot climates. Exercise should be avoided in hot weather, so that problems can be prevented. The dangers of excessive heat are severe heat stroke, which can cause permanent brain damage, seizures, and permanent muscle damage.

Another hazard of exercise is family withdrawal. It is important when people begin to get involved in an exercise program that they maintain a good, healthy perspective on their life. It is important to continue life requirements of family relationships and work requirements so that you aren't totally consumed by an exercise program and withdraw into it.

WHO NEEDS A REGULAR EXERCISE PROGRAM?

Regular exercise is necessary for all people. It is necessary to prevent physical problems, and it is necessary if people already have these problems. In order to prevent serious problems from occurring at a young age, exercise probably should be carried out by all people. The psychological and physical benefits are great. It allows for weight control and keeping one's ideal weight. It can also help with specific medical diseases.

What particular diseases can exercise help? Certainly people with high blood pressure should exercise regularly. It has been well shown that a regular exercise program can decrease blood pressure by 5–10 millimeters of mercury on a regular basis. This, combined with low salt intake and good weight control, may be enough to keep your blood pressure normal. Exercise can also make it unnecessary to take medication to control your blood pressure.

Patients with diabetes on regular exercise programs can help control blood sugar and require less insulin. In people on hemodialysis with chronic renal failure, it has been shown that exercise lowers their triglyceride levels. In addition, the development of atherosclerosis, or hardening of the arteries, is lessened in people who exercise regularly. In people who have had heart attacks or congestive heart failure, exercise can recondition the heart and allow people to enjoy life more fully because they have a better exercise capability; they can walk farther, sleep better at night, and enjoy more activity. A regular exercise program provides the psychological benefit of preventing stress-related diseases such as ulcers and anxiety attacks.

HOW IS AN EXERCISE PROGRAM DETERMINED?

Exercise probably fits into everybody's life in some way or another to benefit any of the conditions mentioned above. Blood tests are used to determine if you need specific exercises and how much exercise to do. All people should have a health assessment made before they start an exercise program. For a person under 25, this can be done by a family member. If you are older than 25 (and certainly for those over 35), a physician should be consulted before starting a regular exercise program, so that a complete examination can be done.

This complete physical examination should include a thorough medical history. In particular, you are looking for history suggestive of heart disease or problems with the lungs or blood vessels. Such conditions as shortness of breath, presence of chest pain, being a smoker or nonsmoker—these determine your exercise capacity. The family history is also important, because if someone has a marked positive family history of problems due to exercise, they may be at risk. Your height and weight should also be determined, so that you have a baseline of numbers to start from to gauge exercise capacity based on your weight. People who are extremely obese should not go out and start running. Nor should people who have been sedentary all their lives; rather, they should start on a slow walking program.

Physical examinations should also include a checking of the blood pressure, listening to the heart and lungs, and examining the peripheral pulses to make sure there is good circulation. Laboratory screening should be done in most, preferably all, people over 35. This should include blood count for anemia, for sugar to rule out the possibility of diabetes, and for cholesterol and triglyceride levels. A urinalysis should be included as a baseline, because sometimes exercise can cause blood urine.

Another necessary test for persons over 35 years old who want to start an exercise program is the baseline electrocardiogram.

Anyone who has these symptoms—chest pains, shortness of breath, and/or lightheadedness and dizziness—should have an exercise tolerance test. Should every person over age 35 have an exercise tolerance test? Yes, if they are going to be involved in a regular, strenuous exercise program. This would mean at least twenty minutes to a half-hour, four to five times per week, of the following activities: running or walking, swimming, bicycling, Nautilus or any of the other exercise machines. Those people should have an exercise test just to assure themselves that they can get their heart rate to a good level and sustain it for an adequate period of time and without any irregular beating of the heart, without any symptoms, and without any sign of marked heart *ischemia*.

The heart rate to shoot for in a regular exercise program is 70 percent of one's maximum heart rate. This 70 percent heart rate should be maintained for approximately twenty minutes. All exercise programs should begin with a five-minute warm up or stretching and gradual buildup of heart rate, and then end with a five-minute cooldown along with postexercise stretching. Maximal heart rate can be estimated by taking 220 and substracting one's age; then 70 percent of this number is considered an ideal heart rate for exercise for cardiac fitness. For example, if a person is 40 years old, 220 minus 40 is 180, and 70 percent of 180 is 126. So a 40-year-old person should attempt to keep his or her heart rate at 126 or thereabouts for twenty minutes to ensure good cardiac condition.

WHAT ARE THE EFFECTS OF EXERCISE AS A PREVENTIVE MEASURE?

Regular exercise has never been shown in an absolutely conclusive, scientifically accepted way to increase your longevity. There is abundant evidence, however, that a regular exercise program will decrease many of the commonly known cardiac risk factors. As mentioned previously, blood pressure may be normalized with regular exercise, weight will be decreased, blood sugar may be normalized and carbohydrate tolerance will be improved. Also, high-density lipoprotein cholesterol (so-called large cholesterol, which is shown to be a protective factor for heart disease) will be increased, triglycerides will be decreased, and people will be less likely to smoke. All these things have been shown to be improvements in known cardiac risk factors. If you are overweight, hypertensive, diabetic with poor glucose control, hyperlipidic, and smoke, your risk of heart disease is markedly increased.

The great benefit of a regular exercise program, then, is that by decreasing these risk factors and normalizing them, a patient's life span will be improved. There is also the psychological benefit of decreasing stress in your life and taking time out for yourself every day. As a result, people have a better outlook on life; they are more relaxed about themselves, they are more satisfied, and they are basically happier; this leads to a better-quality life, if not a longer life.

The benefits of exercise are many, and the risks are extremely few —again, most of the risks can certainly be prevented by using your brain. Problems like muscular/skeletal pains, joint pains, tendinitis, bursitis—all of these can occur from overusing the bones and joints in a regular exercise program. But you can modify your exercise— for instance, following a hard day with an easy day or a day when there is less exercise done. In this way, one takes the easy day to rest the bones and joints, so that most problems can be prevented, or at least minimized.

When one goes into a regular exercise program one has to face the fact that these muscle aches and pains may occur, and not only at the beginning when one is out of condition. They may occur throughout your life, but usually are short-term problems and will not prevent you from exercising completely, although you may have to adjust your exercise to accommodate them. For example, if people have bad arthritis and cannot use their legs, they will have to use their arms for exercise. In some way the heart rate can be increased by good cardiac conditioning.

Heat and dehydration must be avoided. These are things that are easily preventable but can have very serious consequences. The consequences can be muscle damage, brain damage, seizures, potential kidney damage, and even death in rare cases. These things can be easily prevented by drinking adequate fluids before, during, and after exercise, avoiding very hot times of day, and dressing loosely and comfortably. The rubber suits that people wear to lose weight and sweat a lot should be outlawed. They are very, very dangerous to one's health and merely cause the temperature to rise, making you sweat more and lose body fluids without any major benefit. All these risks can be prevented.

It is possible that sudden death can't be prevented, but people should watch for these symptoms: shortness of breath, lightheadedness, and chest pain. If you develop any of these symptoms while exercising, you should stop, walk, get fluid, get in the shade, and seek some help. You should then certainly see your physician and not continue exercising. Those are the risks of exercising and, again, they can be prevented.

The role of family history is an important one. Family history is one of the risk factors described by the Framingham Study, which longitudinally followed people for long periods of time to see what factors lead to increased heart disease and stroke; a positive family history was one of those factors. Positive family history is something we can't do anything about. However, that is where exercise comes in, because exercise allows us to do something about all the other risk factors: weight control, smoking, blood pressure, blood sugar, and lipids. All those risk factors can be improved with regular exercise; your family history cannot be changed.

Even if your family history is strongly positive, you should certainly see a physician before starting a regular exercise program, for a good examination to rule out the possibility that you have heart disease. You can change these other risk factors, so that the family history is important in designing an exercise program. Ethnic background probably doesn't play a role in determining the exercise needed. Black people are known to have a higher incidence of hypertension, but this is detected by a physical examination. All people should exercise, no matter what race or background. The susceptibility is in designing and figuring out someone's exercise program.

People with the greatest risk of heart disease are the ones that need exercise the most; they should not avoid exercise because they have risk factors. People who have positive family histories and all these other risk factors should be exercising more so as to prevent the possibility of heart disease. It has to be done in a well-designed, graded, slowly increasing, well-controlled fashion, but it can be done and should be done.

WHAT ARE THE CURRENT EXERCISE PLANS FOR MOST PEOPLE?

People should exercise to derive the benefits mentioned earlier, benefits that are both physical and psychological. Everybody needs a regular exercise program to control one's weight. We all overeat in this country; we have diets that are much too high in fats. It is important that we get these things under control, keeping blood pressure down, keeping stress to a minimum, and allowing some time in the day to fulfill some inner needs. All these things can be accomplished with a regular exercise program, three times per week. I think that the benefits far outweigh the risks because the risks could be prevented and the benefits are potentially great.

What would be a specific exercise plan?

Most people are advised to start on exercise plans that are aerobic in nature. This means that you are using oxygen all the time that you are exercising. Aerobic types of exercise are walking, running, swimming, bicycling—basically exercise where you can talk all the time. Anaerobic exercise, on the other hand, is weight lifting such that you cannot talk, where you are expelling or holding your breath.

Cardiac benefit is obtained from aerobic conditioning, where you are continuously using oxygen, and the heart is pumping in a regular but fast fashion for a period of time. Start out three to four times per week at the minimum; if you can do more, fine. Start out expecting to do a half-hour program. This should be in addition to any exercise you do at work, because what you have been doing at work is usually not enough. This thirty-minute exercise period should include stretching, mild calisthenics at the beginning, and then five minutes of warmup, whether bicycling, running, walking, or swimming. After five minutes of slow, gradual increasing exercise, do twenty minutes of concerted exercise at 70 percent of your maximum heart rate. This is then followed by five minutes of cooldown, where you are slowing either your walking or your running, and then stretching afterward.

It is extremely important to take plenty of fluids before, some mild fluid during, and then fluid after this type of exercise. The best fluid is water only. Doing exercise for twenty minutes or half an hour, you don't require any sugar or electrolyte replacement, and water is really the best thing you can drink. You should avoid salt replacement; you do not require salt during exercise for this short period of time. You really only require water.

For people who are on medication, it is important to discuss the exercise program with your physician. Dosages of insulin, blood pressure medication, and heart medication (digitalis) can all be affected by exercise. It is important that the dosage and the timing be checked by the physician prior to beginning an exercise program. For example, with insulin, exercise can make the blood sugar go down if it is over a long period to time. You should probably wait to take it until after you exercise, if you exercise in the morning. If you are exercising in the afternoon and you are on insulin in the morning, remember to make sure you take some sugar before and after you exercise, so that the sugar does not get too low. With someone on insulin, blood sugar should probably be checked before, during, and after a regular exercise program; this might possibly be checked while the patient is having an exercise tolerance test.

It is important when designing a specific exercise to pick the correct time of day. Different people have different biological rhythms. Some people like to exercise in the morning, and some people would rather exercise late in the afternoon or evening. For some of us it depends on our work schedules. There are many things that go into a specific schedule but everybody can figure out some time of day to fit in their exercise. Many people exercise at lunchtime, taking the half hour or hour to go out exercising, then eating a smaller lunch at a time when this can be done.

You have to be careful of the heat in certain seasons and certain environments. The clothes that you wear are important. Most exercising requires very minimal equipment, but the equipment you have should be good equipment, so as to prevent injury. For example, if you are walking or running, you need good, comfortable, well-built, well-supported shoes. You also need cool, comfortable clothing. The same thing is true with bicycle riding, swimming, etcetera—whether or not you need goggles and bathing caps, and whether certain types of suits may be more comfortable.

As you go through and maintain your exercise program, you will get tips from other people who are doing the same exercise about exactly what kind of equipment may be good for you. Other good sources of information are the various sporting goods stores, where there may be a person who is well versed in a particular exercise to advise you.

WHAT TYPE OF EXERCISE SHOULD PEOPLE START WITH?

For people who have done no exercise at all, a walking program is recommended: twenty minutes to half an hour, three to four times a week, of good quick walking. You can look around, you can enjoy nature, you can breathe the fresh air, you can chat with somebody you are walking with, you can listen to your Walkman if you like, but it has to be good concerted walking: not window-shopping, not slow walking. You should basically work up a sweat and get your heart rate up to derive benefit from the exercise.

What are other good types of exercise?

Bicycling is a terrific exercise. It can be done outdoors in the spring, summer, and fall, and indoors in the winter with a stationary bike or an attachment to your bike. Rowing is an extremely good exercise both in the water and indoors on various types of rowing machines or other exercise machines. Jogging has been very popular, an extremely good form of cardiac fitness, although people have to be careful of their bones and joints and avoid too much heat; it is an exercise you should build up to very slowly and gradually.

Swimming is a very good exercise, aerobic in nature, with continuous good muscle use and good pulse rate. It can be done throughout the year—outside in the summer, inside in the winter—and can be a very pleasant form of family exercise. What about sports such as basketball, raquetball, and tennis? These are not usually recommended to people as cardiac conditioning exercises, because physical benefits require the twenty minutes to half-hour of good rapid pulse and, again, working up a sweat. Basketball, tennis, and raquetball require short bursts of energy and short bursts of rapid heart rate but not a sustained heart rate. These types of sports are very good when someone is in condition already, but they are not particularly recommended to people who are starting to condition themselves. Those sports can be used in conjunction with a running, walking, or swimming program.

WHAT TYPE OF EXERCISE STRATEGY HELPS PATIENTS AT RISK?

People who have muscular/skeletal injuries (arthritis included) need to be very careful. You need to consult with your physician initially to devise a specific program that will gain cardiac and metabolic improvement without putting your bones, joints, and muscles at risk. It is important that you start out very slowly and build up gradually. You can't be expected to go out and run ten miles the first day. Every three to four weeks, adjustments should be made. Start at the minimum, and then after three or four weeks of doing this, when you can do the activity comfortably, then build up slowly. It is important that someone has good equipment. In order to prevent injuries, stretch before and after exercise, maintain good fluid intake, and get good shoes if you are running or walking. Using your brain as well as your body will allow your body to heal and rest on some days and work hard on other days.

CAN EXERCISE DECREASE CANCER RISK?

In people who already have cancer, although exercise doesn't play much of a role in curing a specific cancer, it can make them feel better. It may give them psychological benefits, depending on what sort of cancer and whether it is in remission or not. This idea was recently tested by a gold medalist Olympic wrestler who had Hodgkin's disease, which was cured.

Exercise may do a few things to prevent cancer. The evidence is hazy and not very scientifically based, but may be helpful. One, exercise will usually decrease people's drive to smoke, so that with less smoking there may be less lung cancer. It will decrease weight; it will normalize the bowels and change one's diet. There is some suggestion that high-fat, high-protein intake, which leads to slow bowel movements or frequent constipation, may also lead to increased risk of bowel cancer. People who exercise regularly usually have very regular, frequent bowel movements and may shift their diet to higher carbohydrate, lower-fat, lower-protein diets, thereby "possibly" helping to prevent cancer.

On G.I. disorders, again, regular exercise may help regulate the bowel and thereby decrease constipation. In people who have irritable bowel syndrome or colitis, it will decrease stress and decrease weight. If you are going to need an operation, if you can get your weight down with exercise, it may certainly speed your recovery.

People with respiratory disease need to be very careful when they begin exercise programs. Respiratory disease of a chronic nature, such as chronic obstructive pulmonary disease, may lead to irregular heart rhythms. Any patient with respiratory disease should certainly have a good exercise tolerance test, performed on a treadmill while monitoring the cardiac rhythm for any signs of ischemia, prior to beginning an exercise program. Asthma may be worsened by exercise in some patients but may be improved in others. Everybody with asthma and with serious lung disease should check first with a physician, and have an exercise test so that the effect of the exercise can be assessed in a controlled environment.

CONSUMER ORGANIZATIONS

There are several. For running there is the American Medical Joggers Association, based in California, and the National Joggers Association. A physician who exercises is a good referral source and a good person to ask. There are many new sports conditioning and sports medicine centers at the major universities, and these are good places to consult in designing an exercise program.

Community centers are often good. YMCAs, Jewish Community Centers, and various other community centers may have an exercise fitness program, or programs where evaluations can be done. Local running clubs are frequently advertised in the newspapers, and there are sporting goods stores where young people who may be involved in regular exercise of various sorts may be a good initial referral source. These places should not be the final referral source, but they may be places where people can go to find out about a physician that is known in the community, about specific equipment that is used, or good places to jog.

Exercise is beneficial for everybody in some way or another, whether it is a psychological benefit or physical benefit. All people can and should do some form of exercise. People over 35 should have a complete physical examination, and anybody with any sign or symptom of a medical problem should have a full exercise tolerance test, electrocardiogram, and complete examination prior to beginning a regular exercise program. Exercise is good for people, and the benefits far outweigh the risks or hazards. These can be prevented by a sane exercise program: taking adequate fluids, dressing properly, and exercising at the proper time of day. The other important strategy is resting one day and working the next.

Do You Have an Allergy?

Currently it is estimated that one in every three Americans—or 75 million people—suffer an allergic reaction of some sort. Many people are unaware they are even experiencing an allergic reaction. The following section provides some guidelines for distinguishing allergic reactions.

HEADACHES

Certain types of headaches, such as migraines, may be triggered by allergens (substances that provoke an allergic reaction). Allergens found in chocolate, cheeses, red wine, smoked meats, and many other foods have been known to cause severe headaches. A way to determine if an allergen may be causing your headache is to keep a record of when the headaches strike, and what type of foods or activities preceded the headache's onset. With this log, you and your doctor may be able to establish a list of certain foods that you should avoid.

A headache that is worse in the morning but improves rapidly when you sit up is probably *not* an allergic reaction, nor are headaches accompanied by a stiff neck and fever, or loss of muscle control (especially in the bladder or anal sphincter).

VISION

Certain foods, odors, and even geographical locations may cause changes in your vision. As with headaches, it is important to note when and where these changes occurred.

Symptoms such as rapid deterioration of vision, loss of vision in one or both eyes, double vision when looking to the extreme left or right, yellowness in the eyes, pain or swelling in one eye only, and unequal size of the pupils are probably *not* caused by an allergic reaction.

HEARING

An unexplained ringing or buzzing sound in your ears may be an allergic reaction. Also, recurrent ear infections, blocked ears, itching in the ear, sounds too loud or soft, and intermittent loss of hearing may be precipitated by an allergen.

However, symptoms such as pain in one ear only, infection accompanied by fever and/or pain and swelling below or behind the ear, deafness, vertigo, nausea, and a tendency to fall in one direction are *not* usually caused by an allergic reaction.

NOSE

Symptoms of an allergic reaction may be a thin, clear discharge from the nose, sneezing fits, and an itchy nose, eyes, or palate.

But a thick, yellowish discharge from the nose usually means that you are suffering from an infection and not an allergy.

MOUTH AND THROAT

Some symptoms of an allergic reaction in your mouth or throat might be a chronic sore throat with no known causes, a constantly dry mouth, difficulty in swallowing, sudden change of voice, or a chemical taste in your mouth.

Symptoms that are probably *not* the result of an allergic reaction are a sore throat accompanied by a fever, a lump in the throat, a persistent cough, chronic sores on the tongue, and a gradual change in your voice. These may be symptoms of other chronic or internal illness. You may require a more thorough physical exam for a diagnosis.

STOMACH

Temporary or constant diarrhea and bloating after meals may result from an allergic reaction.

However, symptoms such as blood in the stool, pain that starts below the breastbone and radiates to the back or to the right of the ribcage, severe pain, or pain that starts at the navel and descends to the lower right stomach are usually *not* caused by an allergic reaction.

SKIN

A red, itchy rash is usually symptomatic of an allergy, while a rash with yellow discharge or pus is not commonly associated with an allergy. "Hives," which are red, raised, itchy bumps, can be caused by shellfish allergy, anxiety, or unknown causes, appearing or disappearing rapidly. Other red, itchy, scaly rashes may be caused by drugs, detergents, or other contact allergens.

TWENTY-TWO

Preventive Dentistry

While good oral hygiene will not, of course, help you live longer, it will make your life considerably more enjoyable. Anyone who has ever experienced the pain and stress caused by a root canal will testify to this. As *The Journal of the American Dental Association* states, most dental problems result from the failure to comply with one or more of these six steps:

1. Brush and floss your teeth at least once a day.
2. Brush after meals whenever possible.
3. Eat sugar-containing foods only with your meals.
4. Avoid snacks and beverages between meals.
5. Use fluorides daily.
6. Get regular dental checkups.

Unfortunately, many people fail to follow these steps. In fact, tooth decay is the most prevalent disease in the United States other than the common cold.

WHAT CAUSES TOOTH DECAY?

Tooth decay begins with plaque, a sticky, colorless layer of bacteria that is constantly forming in your mouth. Sugar combines with certain bacteria found in plaque to form acids. These acids are held against your tooth by plaque. The acids will then attack your tooth's enamel for a period of twenty minutes. After repeated attacks, the enamel breaks down and becomes decayed. This decay eventually marches toward the center of the tooth, where—left untreated—it reaches the pulp and forms an abscess. When this happens, the tooth becomes very painful and will require root canal (endodontic) treatment or extraction.

THE WARNING SIGNS OF TOOTH DECAY

- Is any tooth sensitive to heat, cold, or sweets?
- Is it painful when you chew?
- Is there swelling or drainage at or below the gumline?
- Are there brown spots on the tooth?
- Do you have persistent pain in your mouth or sinus region?

If you answer yes to any of these questions, chances are you have tooth decay; see your dentist immediately.

Proper brushing and flossing techniques, along with a good diet, will minimize your teeth problems considerably.

THE BEST WAY TO BRUSH YOUR TEETH

Place the head of the toothbrush against your tooth, with the bristles pointed toward the gumline at a 45-degree angle. Move the brush back and forth (*not* up and down) with short, gentle scrubbing strokes. Clean the entire outer, and then inner, surfaces of each tooth, remembering to keep the brush angled toward the gumline. (The inside surfaces of the front teeth will require a gentle up-and-down motion with the toothbrush held lengthwise and tilted vertically.) Keep in mind that brushing your tongue will improve your breath.

Brushing, while very important, will not clean every area. To thoroughly clean your teeth, you must also floss at least once a day.

THE BEST WAY TO FLOSS YOUR TEETH

Break off about 18 inches of dental floss, and wind most of it around one of your middle fingers. Then wind the rest of the floss around the same finger on the opposite hand. Use this finger to take used floss as you proceed. Take about one inch of floss between the thumbs and forefingers of each hand, hold it tightly, and pass it between your teeth with a gentle back-and-forth motion. Never snap the floss into the gums.

When the floss reaches the gumline, curve the floss into a C-shape. Next press the floss into the space between the tooth and gum until you feel resistance. While holding the floss tightly, scrape your tooth gently with the floss. Repeat this process on all other teeth.

Your gums may bleed when flossing for the first few days. However, this bleeding will soon stop as the plaque and bacteria are removed. If bleeding persists, consult your dentist.

Thoroughly brushing and flossing your teeth not only fights tooth decay, but also helps prevent gum (periodontal) disease.

GUM (PERIODONTAL) DISEASE

Unremoved plaque makes your gums swell and bleed easily. This unremoved plaque will harden into a deposit called calculus, or tartar, that forms under the gumline and can be removed only by your dentist or dental hygienist. Gum disease may be present for years without you being aware that you even have the disease. By then your teeth and gums may be seriously damaged.

Bleeding from the gums is not a normal condition; it should warn you that you may be on your way toward gum disease. If this bleeding occurs, or if your gums are red, swollen, and tender, you may have inflamed gums (gingivitis). Inflamed gums, left untreated, may develop into gum disease.

Gum disease may eventually destroy some of the bone which supports your teeth. The teeth may then become loose and fall out. Surgical treatment may be necessary to save your teeth.

WARNING SIGNS OF GUM DISEASE

- Gums that bleed when you brush your teeth.
- Red, swollen, or tender gums.
- Pus that appears between your teeth and gums when the gums are pressed.
- Gums that have pulled away from your teeth.
- Teeth that become loose, or separate from each other.
- Changes in the way your teeth fit together when you bite.
- Changes in the way partial dentures fit.
- Bad breath.

A Final Word of Encouragement

In this book, we have tried to give you a more concrete estimate of your present and future health than you have ever had. You may be surprised to find that you have a number of risk factors and a high degree of risk for future health problems, even though you feel great today. You may live what you think is a very healthy life-style, yet still have unavoidable risk factors you inherited.

Remember this: There is only so much you can do to preserve your health. Your goal should be to do all that you can, as far as diet and exercise go, as we discussed in these pages. You should maintain contact with a good physician to ensure that any problems that arise will be caught early. We have outlined many clinically sound approaches to risk reduction in this book. It's now up to you to decide how much change you are willing to make and how quickly.

How hard will you find it to make changes in your life? That depends on how directly vulnerable you feel and how you perceive risk. After all, cigarette smoking is, on a day-to-day level, more dangerous than nuclear power, and yet we actually *pay* farmers to plant tobacco. Often people don't change until the risk is apparent to them personally. If your spouse or close friend has a heart attack or develops lung cancer, then you can see firsthand the impact on his or her life. The disease consequences of health behavior are immediately apparent. As soon as one of my patients has a heart attack or any other serious illness, all the denial and rationalizations go right out the window. Smoking cessation, weight loss, and exercise are easy to do—*after the fact!* My hope is that this book will help you change *before* the problems appear.

One way to sustain momentum after you have made the life-style changes is to find out how much you've improved after you've reduced your risk. Write to General Health Inc. (see the opening pages of this book) for another *Beat the Odds Health Questionnaire* and repeat the whole process four to six months later. Have new blood chemistries drawn, and fill out the new questionnaire.

Another way to reinforce your need for improvement once you've changed is to review your *Beat the Odds Health Profile* with your family physician. If you have certain problems such as high blood pressure, high cholesterol, or diabetes, then it's likely other members of your family are at risk, too. Have them review the *BTO Profile,* and let them benefit from the suggestions in *Beat the Odds.*

When you read your *BTO Profile,* you may find that you frequently have "average" as your risk factor value. In fact, you may be "average" in many categories because that's the way statistics often work out for most people. *But remember:* Average doesn't mean "excellent," or that your "attainable" goal has been reached! The "average" American is much more likely to die of a heart attack than people in many, many other countries. The "average" American's cholesterol is probably 40 points higher than it could be with attention to diet and physical exercise. So try for the "attainable" levels in your *BTO Profile*—don't be satisfied with "average."

What happens if your *BTO Profile* says "you are healthy and have attained all you can." Well, congratulations. But remember, you've reached that point because you lead a healthful life-style. Don't quit just because you are doing well now. Good health behavior is a way of life forever. You also may want to take this test again in a year, just to make sure you're on target.

We have tried, in this book, to give you the positive steps you can take to reduce risk. We've tried, in the face of the serious risks our life-style has given us, to be positive. Our message is to take charge of your health *now.* Don't wait, because you can play a major role in determining your life expectancy. We hope that you will gain from reading this book, take charge of your health, and *beat the odds!*

INDEX

About the Authors

HAROLD S. SOLOMON is forty-five years old and lives in suburban Boston with his wife, Lois, and his teenaged children, Lara and Jeremy. He is currently assistant professor of medicine at Harvard Medical School, where he has been for seventeen years. He is on the staffs of Brigham and Women's Hospital and Beth Israel Hospital in Boston. He devotes most of his professional time to the clinical practice of medicine, specializing in the treatment of hypertension and other preventable risk factors for premature heart attack and stroke. He serves as a curriculum advisor to Harvard medical students and teaches on the wards of the Brigham and Women's Hospital and in the lecture halls of Harvard Medical School. He has served as a consultant to the medical products industry and has published numerous scientific articles about hypertension, as well as several articles and books for the lay public.

He was born in Savannah, Georgia, was graduated from the University of Georgia in chemistry, and received his M.D. degree from the Medical College of Georgia in 1965. He served as senior assistant resident in medicine, then research fellow in medicine at Peter Bent Brigham Hospital from 1969 to 1972. Since 1972 he has been on the full-time staff of Brigham and Harvard Medical School, usually in some role related to hypertension. He served as director of the Hypertension Education Project from 1975 to 1978, studying health motivation techniques.

Dr. Solomon is a Fellow of the American College of Physicians and a member of Alpha Omega Alpha Honor Medical Society.

LAWRENCE D. CHILNICK is an author, medical writer, editor, and book producer specializing in the interpretation of medical and scientific information for consumer and professional audiences.

He is the creator and editor-in-chief of *The Pill Book,* the number-one consumer prescription drug handbook, with more than two and a half million copies in print. He has also created the Pill Book Library, *The Coke Book, The Good News About Depression, The Food Book, Wonder Drugs, Healthy Kids for Life* and *Drugs in the Workplace,* a combined video/print program. He is cocreator of the Audio Health Library, a series of dramatic audio productions on common health problems.

Mr. Chilnick is also an award-winning journalist whose articles have appeared in national medical publications. He lives with his wife, Janet, and two children, Susanna and Jeremy, in New York City.